Diverticulitis Cookbook

The Comprehensive Guide to Delicious and Healing Recipes for 1500+ Days and Easy-to-Follow Recipes to Manage and Prevent Flare-Ups

Carolyn S. Hart

To you, the amazing person who have chosen to buy this **"Diverticulitis Cookbook"** by **Carolyn S. Hart,** I want to express my heartfelt gratitude and appreciation. Your decision to explore this cookbook is not just a purchase; it's a commitment to your health and well-being, and it fills my heart with joy to know that I can be a part of your journey.

I crafted this cookbook with love, passion, and a deep understanding of the challenges faced by those dealing with diverticulitis. Each recipe is more than just a collection of ingredients; it's a flavorful expression of care and nourishment, carefully designed to support your dietary needs while delighting your taste buds.

When you open the pages and discover the mouthwatering dishes waiting to be savored, I hope you feel a sense of excitement and anticipation. From hearty soups to vibrant salads, comforting casseroles to wholesome snacks, every recipe is a celebration of wholesome ingredients and mindful cooking.

As you begin on this culinary adventure, I encourage you to savor each moment in the kitchen, relish the aromas that fill your home, and indulge in the flavors that bring joy to your palate. Cooking and enjoying meals should be a source of pleasure and gratitude, and I hope this cookbook brings both into your life.

Thank you for choosing the **"Diverticulitis Cookbook by Carolyn S. Hart."** Your purchase means the world to me, and I am deeply grateful for the opportunity to be a part of your health and wellness journey. Here's to delicious meals, vibrant health, and moments of culinary bliss shared with loved ones. Cheers to you and happy cooking!

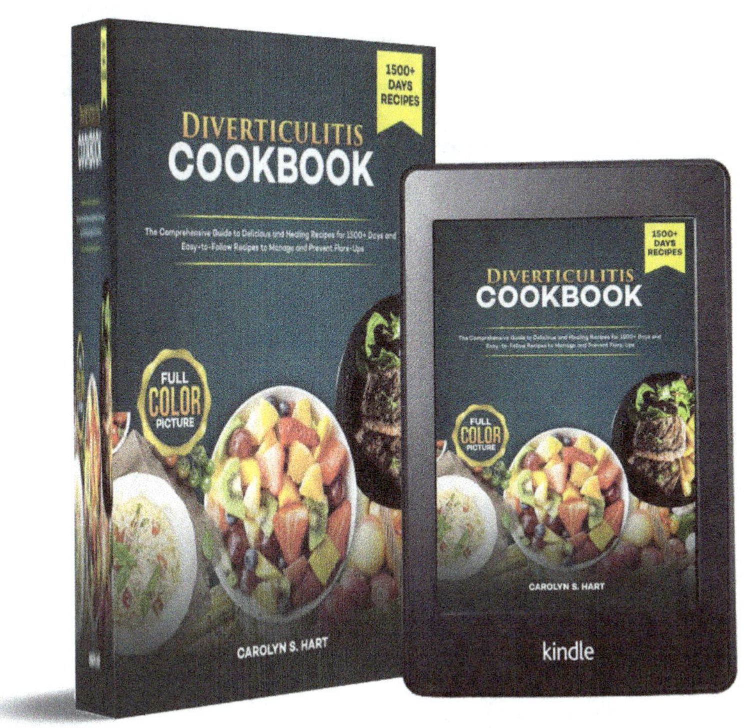

COPYRIGHT © 2024 [CAROLYN S. HART]

TABLE OF CONTENTS

HOW THIS COOKBOOK CAN HELP YOU

This cookbook aims to provide people with diverticulitis with simple and convenient recipe ideas that can help prevent and manage their symptoms. As the book will outline, a combination of medical intervention and small lifestyle changes, such as incorporating certain ingredients into your diet, can make a big difference when it comes to reducing the discomfort of diverticulitis. However, knowing where to start with such big lifestyle changes can be challenging, and it can be tempting in the spur of the moment.

This book will give people with diverticulitis access to innovative, healthy and nutritious meal ideas suitable for all tastes and mealtimes that will provide readers with both inspiration and a way to manage their symptoms.

Every recipe you'll find in these pages has been designed and created specifically for you, along with the recipe title and the dish's ingredients and method, each recipe features: an explanation of how you can incorporate that dish into a weekly meal plan to keep your meals varied and interesting, estimated calories per serving so you can stay on top, your daily intake for a healthy, balanced diet, and an indication of what type of meal the dish is suitable for, for example, whether it's a quick lunch fix or a more leisurely dinner.

Enjoy the recipes and good luck!

INTRODUCTION

Dear Reader,

Have you ever witnessed a friend's struggle and felt an overwhelming desire to make a difference in help them? That's exactly how this cookbook came to life – through a journey of compassion, friendship, and a shared determination to overcome health challenges.

Let me introduce you to my friend Laurel, a dear friend whose battle with diverticulitis and this sparked a culinary revolution in my lives. Like many others facing this condition, Laurel experienced painful flare-ups that disrupted her daily routines and brought moments of discomfort. So I determination to support her on this journey, I embarked on a mission to create recipes that not only nourished her body but also brought joy to her meals.

In the process, I discovered a world of flavors, ingredients, and cooking techniques that not only supported Laurel's digestive health but also delighted her taste buds. From comforting soups that soothed her during tough times to vibrant salads that celebrated the goodness of fresh produce, each recipe was a labor of love and a testament to our shared commitment to wellness.

As Laurel found healing and relief through these flavorful creations, I realized that our journey could benefit others facing similar challenges. And thus, the "Diverticulitis Cookbook" was born – a collection of recipes infused with care, expertise, and the desire to empower individuals on their path to digestive wellness.

So, as you turn the pages and explore the culinary delights within, know that you're not just buying a cookbook – you're embarking on a journey of healing, discovery, and a celebration of good food shared with loved ones.

Welcome to the "Diverticulitis Cookbook." You will find recipes that will nourish your body, uplift your spirit, and bring moments of joy to your kitchen table.

Carolyn S. Hart.

CHAPTER 1

WHAT IS DIVERTICULITIS?

Have you ever felt a sudden sharp pain in the lower left side of your abdomen? This symptom may be due to bloating, constipation or a change in your bowel habits. If so, you may think you may have diverticulitis. This chapter explains this digestive condition in detail so you can properly manage your gut health.

Imagine the giant intestine, also called the colon, as a long muscular tube charged with absorbing water and electrolytes from digested food waste. In a healthy colon, the lining is easily aligned. However, in diverticulosis, small pouches or bulges, known as diverticula, expand in the weakened outer wall of the colon. These bags are usually formed in areas where blood vessels penetrate the colon wall.

Although diverticulosis itself is usually harmless and often ignored, some people develop inflammation or infection in one or more of these diverticula. This condition is known as diverticulitis and can cause severe pain.

UNDERSTANDING THE DIFFERENCE: DIVERTICULOSIS VS DIVERTICULITIS

Consider diverticulosis as a precursor to diverticulitis. Here's a breakdown of the major changes:

- **Diverticulosis:** the presence of pouches (diverticules) in the wall of the large intestine, but often there are no symptoms.
- **Diverticulitis:** inflammation or infection of one or more diverticula. It causes pain, sensitivity and other digestive problems.

RISK FACTORS AND CAUSES OF DIVERTICULITIS

Although the exact cause of diverticulitis remains unknown, many factors are thought to increase the risk.

- **Age:** Diverticulitis is not uncommon in people over 40 years of age.
- **Diet:** Bottom line: A low-fiber diet without vegetables and whole grains can lead to diverticulosis, which then turns into diverticulitis.
- **Obesity:** Excess weight puts pressure on your digestive system.
- **Lack of Exercise:** Regular physical activity promotes intestinal health and reduces the risk of diverticulitis.
- **Smoking:** Smoking weakens the walls of your colon and can lead to infection.
- **Certain Medications:** Corticosteroids and some nonsteroidal anti-inflammatory drugs (NSAIDs) may increase your risk.

SYMPTOMS OF DIVERTICULITIS:

Diverticulitis can cause headaches if left untreated, so it's important to seek medical care right away if you experience any of the following symptoms.

Common signs and symptoms include:

- Sudden severe pain with a decrease in the left side of the abdomen (although the location of the pain may be different)
- Reduction of stomach sensitivity
- Feeling bloated
- Change in bowel behavior (constipation or diarrhea)
- Nausea
- Heat
- Shivering

UNDERSTAND YOUR ROLE IN THE MANAGEMENT OF DIVERTICULITIS

Your life should not be limited by the prognosis of diverticulitis. This book will be your companion on your journey to gut fitness. In later chapters, you will discover the nutritional steps encouraged for diverticulitis, delicious, gut-friendly recipes designed for each stage, and the different nutritional steps encouraged for social gatherings.

Tips for maintaining a healthy lifestyle with the right knowledge and dietary approach, you can reverse diverticulitis and enjoy a fulfilling life.

FOODS TO INCLUDE IN YOUR DIET

The foods you should include in your diverticulitis diet depend on the specific stage you are at. Here is a summary of the recommended ingredients for each section:

CLEAR LIQUID DIET (FOR FLARE-UPS):

This short-term diet plan is designed to rest the digestive system and fight infections. Focus on clean drinks that hydrate and minimize stress on digestion. Some examples are:

- **Water:** essential for hydration.
- **Clear Soup or Broth:** provides electrolytes and heat.
- **Decaffeinated Tea or Coffee:** provides some relaxation, but limits the laxative effects of consumption.
- **Strained Apple or Cranberry Juice**: provides some nutrients and hydration, but is limited by its sugar content.
- **Ice Cream or Ice Chips:** Soothes a sore throat and keeps you hydrated.

LOW RESIDUAL DIET (FOR RECOVERY):

Once symptoms return, you can switch to a low-residue diet. This diet includes foods that are easily digestible and have minimal impact on the digestive system.

The content is as follows:

- **Refined Grains:** In this section, white bread, white rice, and soft pasta are easier to digest than whole grains.
- **Lean Protein Sources:** Skinless, baked cookies, fish, and eggs are easy on your gut.
- **Low-Fiber Vegetables:** Choose properly cooked vegetables without skin or seeds. This includes beans, carrots and potatoes.
- **Low-Fiber Fruits:** Canned or cooked fruits without skin or seeds (applesauce, pears, peaches) contain important vitamins.
- **Yogurt (plain, low-fat):** A good source of probiotics that may improve gut health.
- **Cottage Cheese:** Provides protein and a small amount of calcium.

HIGH-FIBER MAINTENANCE DIET (FOR LONG-TERM PREVENTION):

After recovery from a flare-up, a high-fiber weight loss program is essential for long-term gut health and can possibly prevent further problems. The nutritional needs of this section are:

- **Fruits**: (fresh, frozen or canned): Different end results provide essential vitamins, minerals and fiber.
- **Vegetables:** Choose a variety of vegetables including leafy greens, broccoli, Brussels sprouts, and squash.
- **Whole Grains:** Brown rice, quinoa, oats, and oats are excellent sources of fiber and important nutrients.
- **Beans and Legumes:** Lentils, peas and black beans are rich in fiber and protein. However, introduce it steadily to avoid excess gas.
- **Nuts and seeds (in moderation):** Provide healthy fat and fiber, but understand the portion sizes.
- **Lean Protein Sources:** If you want to get your protein, still eat chicken, fish or tofu.

FOODS TO AVOID

Although there is no list of forbidden foods for diverticulitis, the structures and positive properties of food can stimulate the digestive system, especially during periods of recovery. Here is a summary of the foods you should generally avoid or limit in your diverticulitis diet.

FOODS RICH IN FIBER (DURING THE RECOVERY PERIOD):

- **Whole Grains:** Although essential to a healthy weight loss program, whole grains such as brown rice, quinoa, and whole-wheat bread can be difficult to digest during recovery. Be sure to consistently reintroduce them during high fiber maintenance segments.

- **Nuts, Seeds and Popcorn:** These can be high in fiber and can irritate the digestive system, especially during a flare-up. However, research suggests that it may be safe for a small number of humans in the maintenance phase. Please consult your doctor for individual advice.

- **Fruits and Vegetables Rich in Fiber:** Fruits with pores, skins and seeds (apples, pears, berries) and vegetables such as broccoli, Brussels sprouts and cabbage are rich in fiber and support the digestive system through inflammation and healing. they stimulate There is a possibility. . During the maintenance phase, cooked foods can be reintroduced in small amounts.

- **Beans And Legumes:** While good sources of dietary fiber in a healthy diet, beans and legumes (lentils, chickpeas, black beans) are good for fuel and bloating, especially during flare-ups and recovery. Introduce them periodically during the maintenance phase.

OTHER FOODS TO LIMIT:

- **Red Meat:** it is rich in fat and difficult to digest. Use lean protein sources such as chicken and fish.
- **Processed Meats:** Processed meats such as sausages and bacon are always high in fat, sodium, and nitrates, which can aggravate your digestive system.
- **Spicy Foods:** Spicy foods can irritate the digestive lining and aggravate symptoms during the exacerbation process.
- **Alcohol:** Too much alcohol can cause inflammation and dehydration. Limit or completely avoid alcohol consumption during exacerbation of the disease.
- **Caffeinated Drinks:** Coffee and caffeinated tea also have a laxative effect and can worsen diarrhea. Please limit your intake or consult your doctor.
- **Fizzy Drinks:** Fizzy drinks can cause bloating and gas, especially during certain stages of flare-ups. Use clean water or broth instead.

ADDITIONAL CONSIDERATIONS:

- **FODMAP:** Some studies suggest that a low-FODMAP (restricting positive fermentable carbohydrates) diet may help manage the signs and symptoms of diverticulitis. However, consult your doctor or nutritionist before making any major changes to your diet.
- **Fried Foods:** Fried foods usually contain too much fat and are difficult to digest. Choose healthier cooking methods, such as baking, grilling, and steaming.
- **High-Fat Dairy Products:** High-fat dairy products such as milk, cheese, and ice cream can be difficult to digest, especially during exacerbations. If you're concerned about dairy, choose low-fat or lactose-free alternatives.

CHAPTER 2

ROLE OF FIBER IN DIVERTICULAR HEALTH

Fiber, a word often associated with healthy digestion, can be a little confusing for people with diverticulitis. There are science behind fiber and how it can be your ally in dealing with gut health.

Fiber is not your enemy, but your friend when dealing with diverticulitis. By becoming familiar with the unique types of fiber and gradually including them in your diet, you can strengthen your bowels and reduce the likelihood of relapse.

DIVERTICULITIS AND FIBER

Dietary fiber is an element obtained from plants, but our body cannot fully digest it. There are two important types.

- **Water-Soluble Dietary Fiber:** Dissolves in water and creates a gel-like substance in the intestine. This slows down digestion, promotes satiety, and regulates blood sugar levels.
- **Insoluble Fiber:** Does not dissolve in water, adds volume to the stool, and helps the easy circulation of food in the digestive system.

FIBROUS DIVERTICULITIS

The exact cause of diverticulitis is still unknown, but low-fiber weight loss programs are thought to be a major contributing factor. Here's why:

- **Problems Caused by Lack of Fiber:** Loss of fiber can make stool hard and difficult to pass. This strain compresses the colon septum, possibly contributing to the formation of diverticula (pouches) and increasing the risk of inflammation.
- **The Protective Role OF Fiber:** Excessive fiber consumption produces softer, bulkier stools that can pass through the large intestine without difficulty. This may reduce stress on the colonic septum and reduce the risk of exacerbation of diverticulitis.

BEYOND THE BASICS: DIFFERENT TYPES OF FIBROSIS AND DIVERTICULITIS

All fibers are beneficial, but some types are especially relevant to diverticular health.

- **Soluble Fiber:** Research shows that soluble fiber plays an important role in the fight against diverticulitis. It may improve bowel movements and reduce infections. Examples include psyllium husk (prescribed by dietary supplements) and oatmeal.

- **Insoluble Fiber:** Some studies show that insoluble fiber can worsen digestive distress in the acute phase, but can help improve long-term gut health by promoting regularity and reducing constipation. It may play an important role in your health. Examples include wheat bran and cellulose.

THE IMPORTANCE OF A BALANCED APPROACH

A balanced, supplemental weight loss program that combines soluble and insoluble fiber is important for long-term gut health and can possibly prevent diverticulitis from recurring. However, during flare-ups, your doctor may recommend a short-term low-fiber diet to help calm your digestive system.

FIBER AND YOU: A GRADUAL PROCESS

If you're new to a high-fiber diet, it's important to steadily increase your intake. This allows your gut bacteria to adapt and reduces the risk of gas and bloating.

Below are some suggestions.

- **Start Small:** Start by including small amounts of fiber-rich foods in your diet and gradually increase the amount over several weeks.

- **Adequate Hydration:** When consuming dietary fiber, it is important to drink enough water throughout the day to help it pass through your digestive system easily.

- **Listen To Your Body:** Be curious about how your body reacts to its unique fiber sources. If you experience excessive gas or bloating, change your intake or consult your doctor.

CHAPTER 3

DEALING WITH DIVERTICULITIS

Diverticulitis can be difficult, but it doesn't have to define you. This chapter explores other lifestyle strategies that may work alongside a diet to improve fitness and overall gut health.

BEYOND THE PLATE: ESSENTIAL HABITS FOR A DIVERTICULITIS-FRIENDLY LIFESTYLE

1. **Hydration is Key:** Water is your best friend for gut quality. Try to drink eight glasses of water a day so that your stools are soft and pass easily through the colon.

2. **Maintaining a Healthy Weight:** Excess weight puts pressure on your digestive system. Aim for a healthy weight with a balanced diet and regular exercise.

3. **Exercise:** Regular physical activity promotes bowel movement, which helps relieve constipation. Aim for at least 30 minutes of low-intensity exercise on the longest day of the week.

4. **Manage Stress:** Chronic stress can negatively affect gut health. Consider relaxation techniques such as yoga, meditation, and deep breathing to better manage stress.

5. **Do Not Smoke:** Smoking weakens the walls of the colon, making inflammation worse and possibly making diverticulitis worse. Quitting smoking is one of the biggest things you can do to improve your overall gut health.

6. **Consider Probiotics:** Probiotics are live microorganisms that may benefit your gut microbiome. Research into their effectiveness in treating diverticulitis is ongoing, but some studies suggest they may be helpful. Talk to your doctor about whether probiotics are right for you.

7. **Regular Doctor Visits:** Schedule daily appointments with your doctor to explore your diverticulitis and discuss any problems you may have. Early detection and control of capacity increases are very important.

8. **Build A Support System:** Living with a chronic condition like diverticulitis can be difficult. Don't be afraid to build support, whether it's in your circle of relatives, friends, or referral organizations for people with diverticulitis. It is useful to share your research and learn from others.

PHASE 1
CLEAR LIQUID DIET (FOR FLARE-UPS)

CHAPTER 4

CLEAR LIQUID DIET (FOR FLARE-UPS) RECIPES

CREAMY OATMEAL WITH BANANAS AND ALMONDS

Ingredients:

- 1/2 cup oatmeal
- 1 cup of water or milk (almond milk for the milk-free option)
- 1 ripe banana, sliced
- 2 tablespoons of chopped almonds
- One teaspoon of honey (but optional)

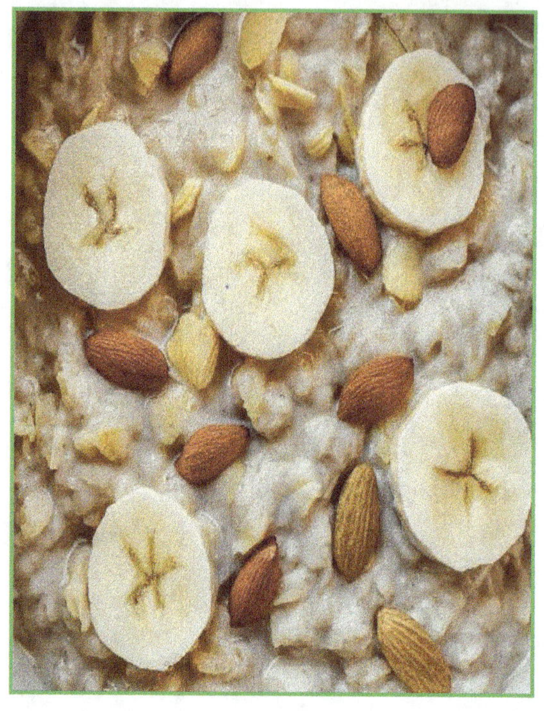

Directions:

1. Bring water or milk to a boil in a saucepan.
2. Add the oatmeal and reduce the heat to low. Cook for 5-7 minutes, stirring occasionally.
3. Once the oats are cooked and creamy, remove from the heat and stir in the sliced bananas and chopped almonds.
4. Drizzle with honey or maple syrup as desired.

Nutritional information:

Calories: 320

Protein: 8 g

Carbohydrates: 52 g

Fiber: 7g

Fats: 10 g

Ingredients:

- 1 cup plain Greek yogurt
- 1/2 cup mixed berries (such as strawberries, blueberries, raspberries)
- 1/4 cup granola (choose low-sugar, high-fiber granola)
- 1 spoon of honey (optional)

Directions:

1. Layer Greek yogurt, blended strawberries and granola in a serving glass or bowl.
2. Drizzle with honey as desired.
3. Serve chilled.

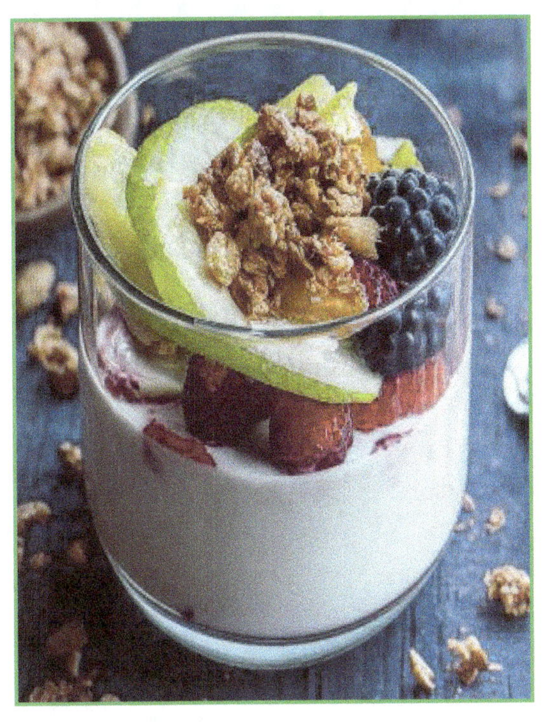

Nutritional information:

Calories: 280

Proteins: 20 g

Carbohydrates: 38 g

Fiber: 6g

Fats: 7 g

Ingredients:

- 1 cup of plain Greek yogurt
- 2 eggs
- 1 cup of fresh spinach leaves
- 1/4 cup crumbled feta cheese
- Salt and pepper to taste
- 1 teaspoon of olive oil

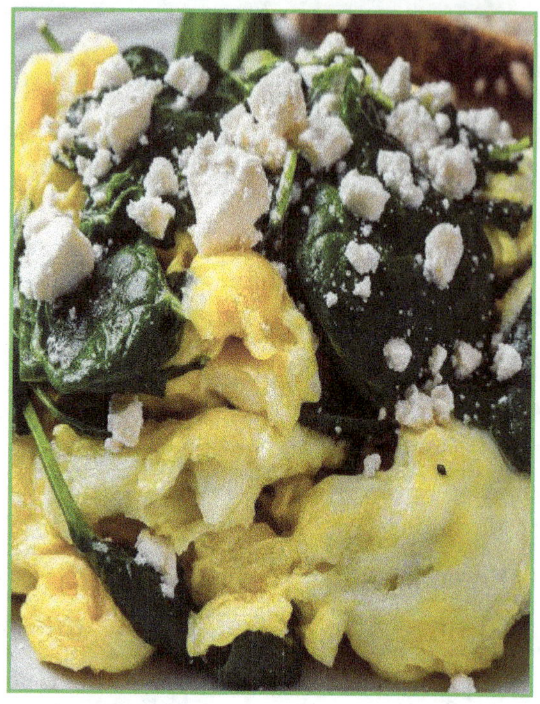

Directions:

1. Heat the vegetable oil in a nonstick pan on medium heat.
2. Add fresh spinach and sauté until wilted.
3. Beat the eggs with salt and pepper in a bowl.
4. Pour the eggs into the pan with the spinach.
5. Cook, stirring gently, until the eggs are scrambled and cooked through.
6. Before serving, sprinkle the scrambled eggs with crumbled feta cheese.

Nutritional information:

Calories: 280

Protein: 18 g

Carbohydrates: 4 g

Fiber: 2g

Fats: 21 g

Ingredients:

- 2 tablespoons of chia seeds
- 1/2 cup of almond milk
- 1/2 teaspoon of vanilla extract
- Fresh fruit for topping (such as sliced strawberries, kiwi or mango)
- 1 tablespoon chopped nuts (optional)

Directions:

1. Mix chia seeds, almond milk and vanilla extract in a bowl. Mix well.
2. Let the mixture sit for 10-15 minutes, stirring occasionally, until it thickens to a pudding-like consistency.
3. Transfer the pudding with chia seeds to a serving bowl and sprinkle with fresh fruit and chopped nuts.
4. Serve chilled.

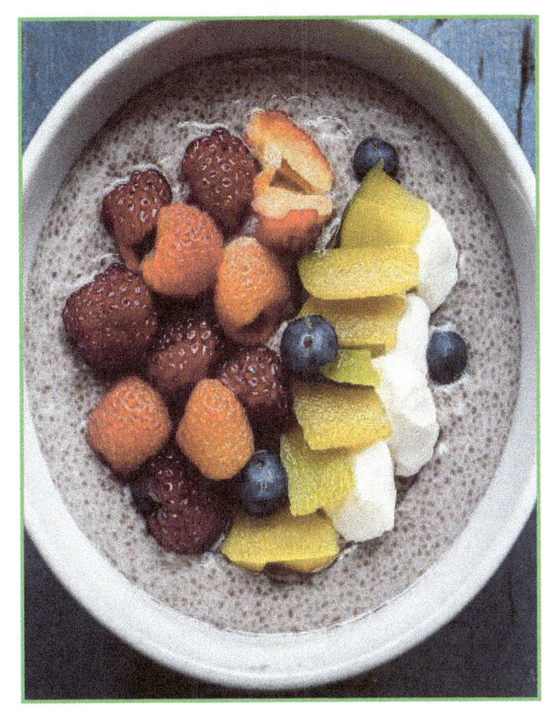

Nutritional information:

Calories: 220

Protein: 5 g

Carbohydrates: 25 g

Fiber: 10g

Fats: 12 g

Ingredients:

- 1 ripe banana
- 1 tablespoon of almond butter
- 1 cup of almond milk
- 1/2 teaspoon of cinnamon
- Ice cubes (optional)

Directions:

1. Combine banana, almond butter, almond milk and cinnamon in a blender.
2. Blend until smooth and creamy.
3. If necessary, add ice cubes and mix again.
4. Pour into a glass and serve immediately.

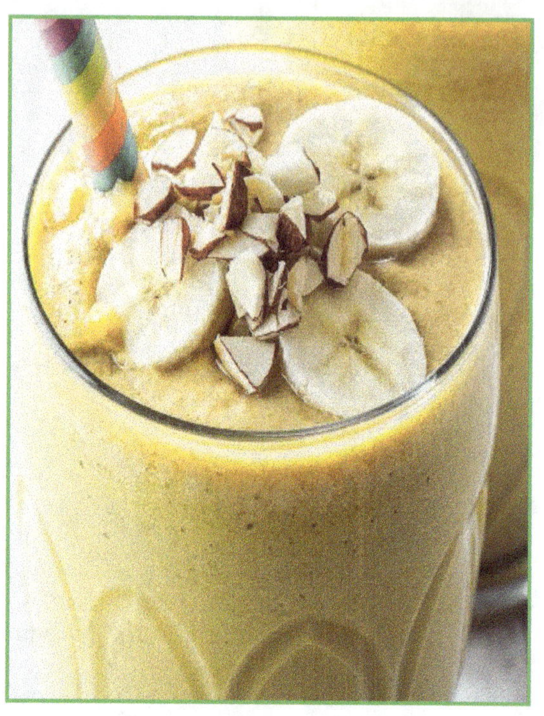

Nutritional information:

Calories: 290

Proteins: 5 g

Carbohydrates: 35 g

Fiber: 6g

Fats: 15 g

Ingredients:

- 4 eggs
- 1 cup of fresh spinach leaves
- 1/2 cup chopped mushrooms
- 1/4 cup chopped onion
- Salt and pepper to taste
- 1 tablespoon of olive oil

Directions:

1. Preheat oven to 350°F (175°C).
2. In an oven-safe pan, heat the olive oil to medium heat.
3. Add diced onion and mushrooms, sauté until soft.
4. Add fresh spinach to pan and cook until wilted.
5. Combine eggs, salt, and pepper and mix in a bowl.
6. Pour the egg mixture over the vegetables in the pan.
7. Cook on the hob for a few minutes until the edges start to set.
8. Transfer the pan to the preheated oven and bake for about 10-12 minutes, or until the frittata is cooked through and set.
9. Slice and serve warm.

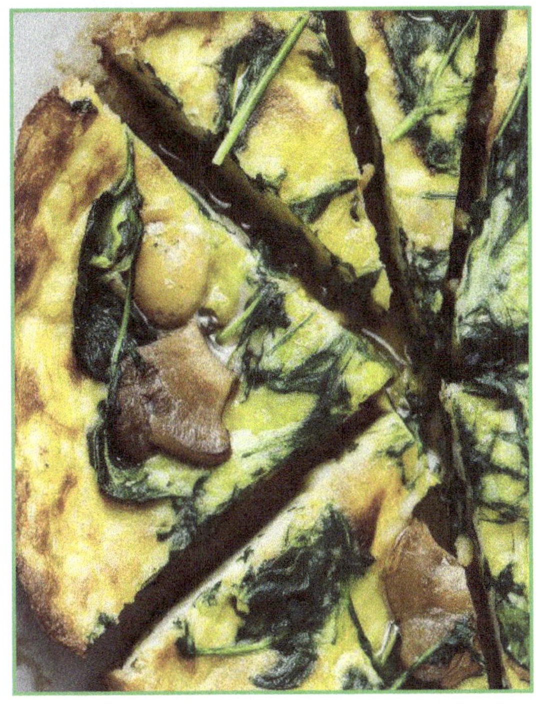

Nutritional information:

Calories: 220

Protein: 14 g

Carbohydrates: 5 g

Fiber: 2g

Fats: 16g

Ingredients:

- 1/4 cup coconut flour
- 2 eggs
- 1/2 cup of almond milk
- 1/2 teaspoon of baking powder
- 1 tablespoon coconut oil (for cooking)
- Fresh strawberries for topping (optional)
- Maple syrup or honey (optional)

Directions:

1. In a bowl, whisk the coconut flour, eggs, almond milk and baking powder until smooth.
2. Heat the coconut oil in a non-stick pan over medium heat.
3. Pour the batter into the pan and make small pancakes.
4. Cook until bubbles form on the surface, then flip and cook until golden brown on both sides.
5. Serve pancakes topped with fresh fruit and drizzled with maple syrup or honey as desired.

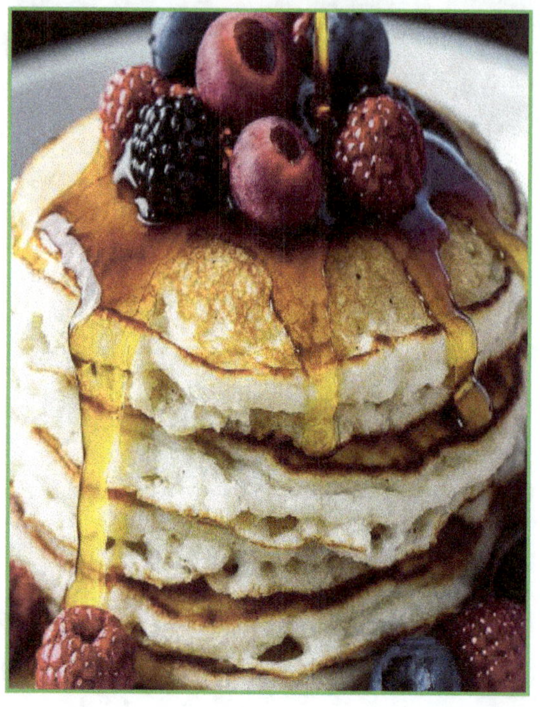

Nutritional information:

Calories: 220

Proteins: 10 g

Carbohydrates: 14 g

Fiber: 6g

Fats: 13g

Ingredients:

- 1 ripe avocado
- 2 slices whole grain bread
- 2 eggs
- Salt and pepper to taste
- 1 tablespoon of vinegar (to poach eggs)
- Fresh herbs for garnish (optional)

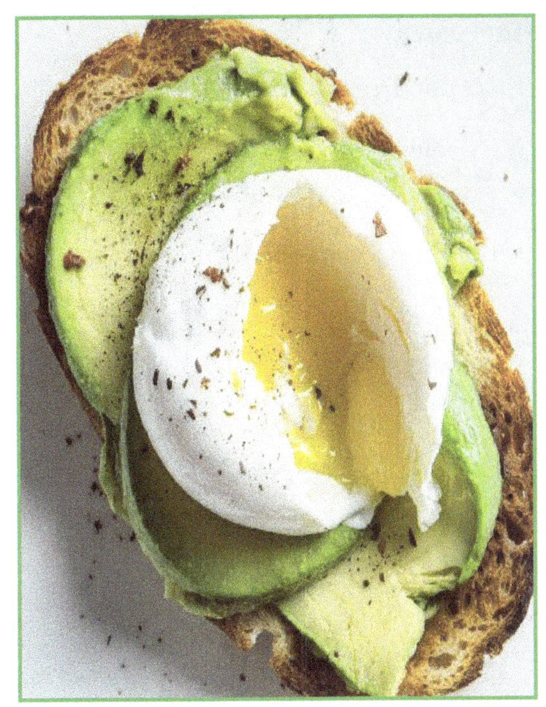

Directions:

1. Toast the whole grain bread till golden brown.
2. While the bread is toasting, prepare the poached eggs. Bring a pot of water to a gentle simmer and add vinegar.
3. Crack each egg into a small bowl or ramekin. Create a whirlpool in the simmering water and gently slide the eggs into the center.
4. Poach the eggs for about 3-4 minutes until the whites are set but the yolks are still runny. Remove with a spoon that is slotted and strain the excess water.
5. Mash the ripe avocado in a bowl and season with salt and pepper.
6. Spread the mashed avocado evenly onto the toasted bread slices.
7. Place a poached egg on top of each avocado toast.
8. Garnish with fresh herbs if desired and serve immediately.

Nutritional information:

Calories: 280

Protein: 14g

Carbohydrates: 25g

Fiber: 10g

Fat: 15g

BLUEBERRY ALMOND SMOOTHIE BOWL

Ingredients:

- 1/2 cup frozen blueberries
- 1/2 banana
- 1/4 cup almond milk
- 1 tablespoon almond butter
- Toppings: sliced almonds, fresh blueberries, granola

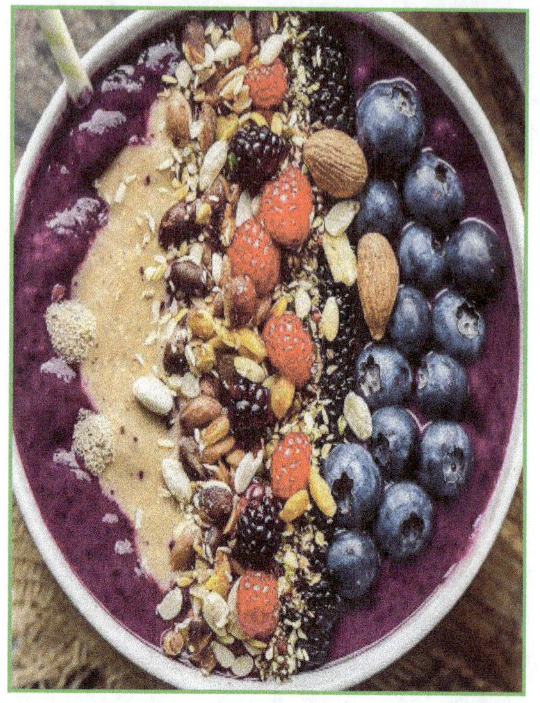

Directions:

1. In a blender, combine frozen blueberries, banana, almond milk, and almond butter.
2. Blend until smooth and creamy.
3. Pour the smoothie into a serving container.
4. Top with sliced almonds, fresh blueberries, and granola.
5. Enjoy with a spoon.

Nutritional information:

Calories: 280

Protein: 8g

Carbohydrates: 35g

Fiber: 8g

Fat: 14g

Ingredients:

- 1 whole grain tortilla
- 2 ounces smoked salmon
- 1/4 avocado, sliced
- 1 tablespoon of cream cheese
- Fresh spinach leaves
- Sliced cucumber (optional)

Directions:

1. Spread Greek yogurt or cream cheese evenly on the whole grain wrap.
2. Layer smoked salmon, avocado slices, fresh spinach, and sliced cucumber (if using) on top of the spread.
3. Roll up the wrap tightly.
4. Cut in half diagonally and serve.

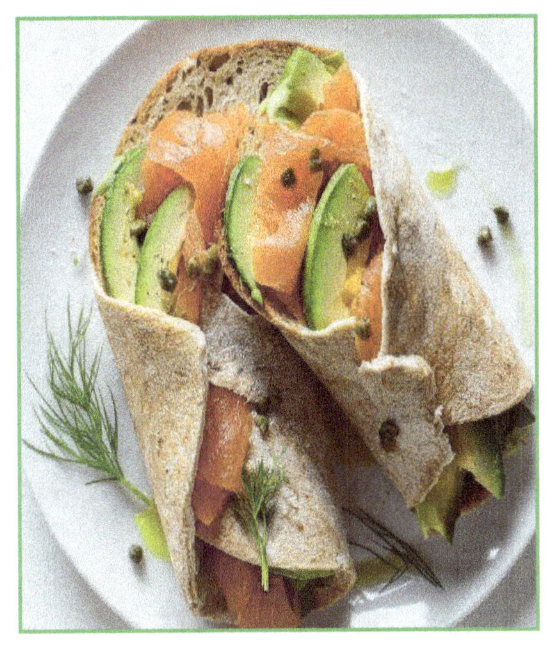

Nutritional information:

Calories: 320

Protein: 20g

Carbohydrates: 25g

Fiber: 8g

Fat: 15g

Ingredients:

- 1 cup rolled oats
- 1 apple, diced
- 1 teaspoon cinnamon
- 1 tablespoon maple syrup
- 1 cup almond milk
- 1 egg for added protein

Directions:

1. Preheat oven to 350°F (175°C). Grease a baking dish.

2. In a bowl, combine rolled oats, diced apple, cinnamon, maple syrup, almond milk, and egg (if using). Mix well.

3. Pour the entire mixture into the already prepared baking dish.

4. Bake for 25-30 minutes or until the top is golden brown and the oats are cooked through.

5. Serve warm, optionally topped with a drizzle of maple syrup or a dollop of Greek yogurt.

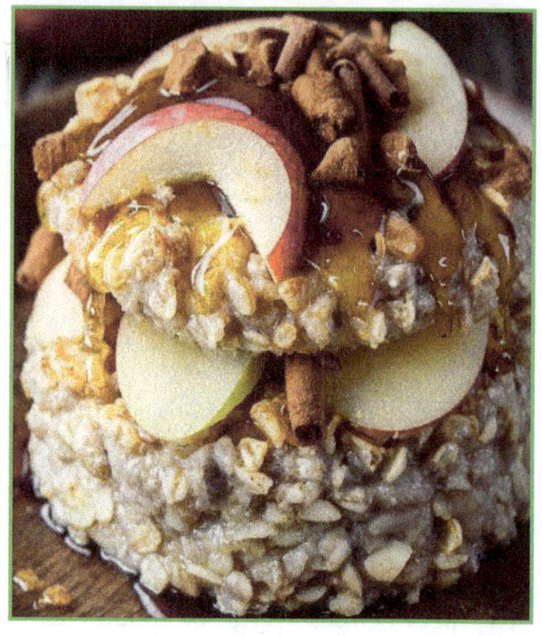

Nutritional information:

Calories: 280

Protein: 8g

Carbohydrates: 40g

Fiber: 6g

Fat: 10g

Ingredients:

- 2 whole grain tortillas
- 1 cup fresh spinach leaves
- 1/2 cup of chopped mozzarella
- 1/4 cup diced tomatoes
- Salt and pepper to taste
- Olive oil for cooking

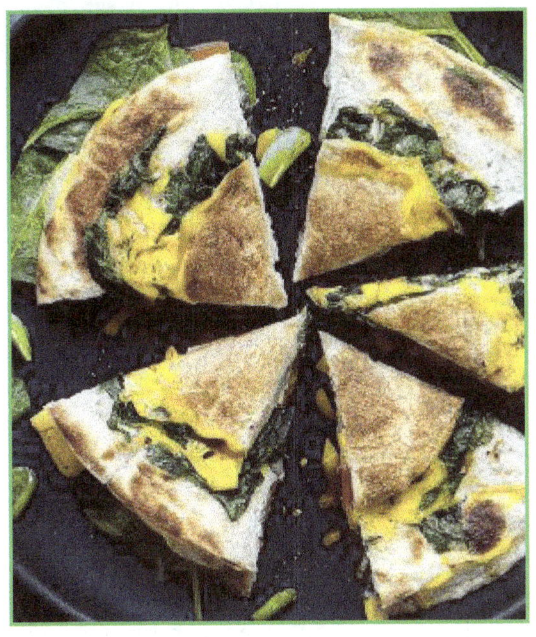

Directions:

1. With medium heat, heat the olive oil in a skillet.
2. Place one tortilla in the skillet and sprinkle half of the shredded cheese evenly over the tortilla.
3. Layer fresh spinach leaves and diced tomatoes on top of the cheese.
4. Season with salt and pepper.
5. Sprinkle the remaining cheese on top and cover with the second tortilla.
6. Cook until the bottom tortilla is golden brown, then carefully flip the quesadilla to cook the other side.
7. Once both sides are crispy and the cheese is melted, remove from heat and let cool slightly before slicing into wedges.
6. Serve warm.

Nutritional information:

Calories: 320

Protein: 15g

Carbohydrates: 25g

Fiber: 6g

Fat: 18g

Ingredients:

- 1/2 cup rolled oats
- 1/2 cup almond milk
- 1 tablespoon peanut butter
- 1/2 banana, mashed
- 1 teaspoon chia seeds (optional)
- Honey or maple syrup for sweetness (optional)

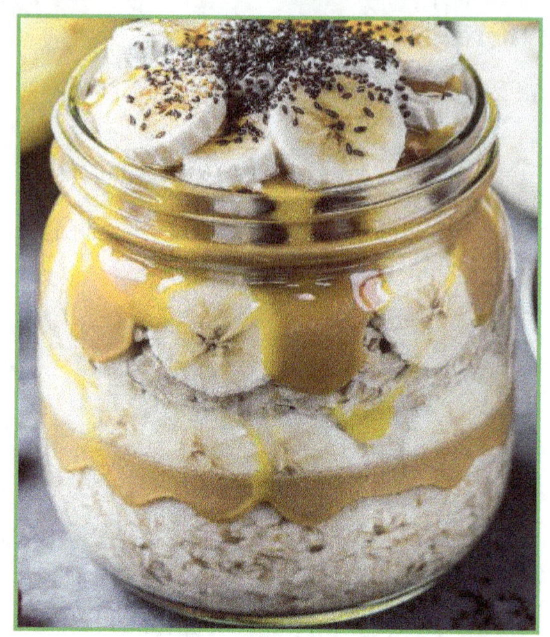

Directions:

1. In a jar or container, combine rolled oats, almond milk, peanut butter, mashed banana, and chia seeds (if using). Stir well.

2. Cover the container and chill for at least 4 hours.

3. Before serving, stir the overnight oats and add honey or maple syrup for sweetness if desired.

4. Enjoy cold or warm it up in the microwave before eating.

Nutritional information:

Calories: 320

Protein: 10g

Carbohydrates: 45g

Fiber: 8g

Fat: 12g

Ingredients:

- 1 whole grain wrap
- 2 eggs, scrambled
- 2 slices turkey breast
- 1/4 avocado, sliced
- Fresh spinach leaves
- Salsa or hot sauce (optional)

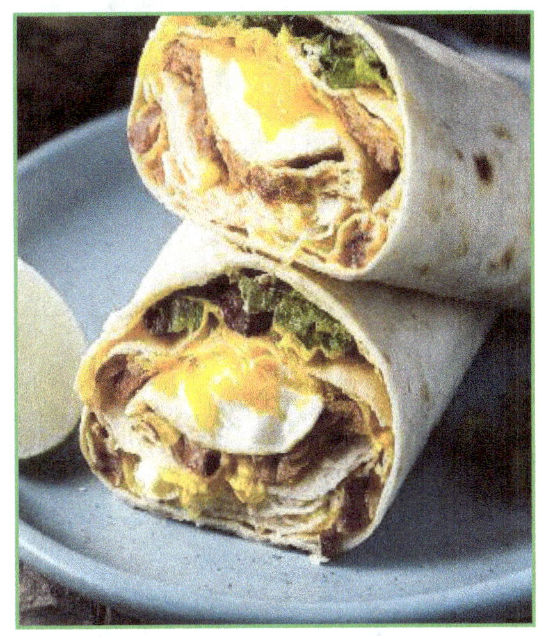

Directions:

1. Warm the whole grain wrap or tortilla in a skillet or microwave.
2. Layer scrambled eggs, turkey slices, avocado slices, fresh spinach leaves, and salsa or hot sauce (if using) on the wrap.
3. Roll up the burrito tightly, tucking in the sides as you roll.
4. Slice the burrito in half diagonally if desired and serve.

Nutritional information:

Calories: 320

Protein: 20g

Carbohydrates: 25g

Fiber: 8g

Fat: 15g

Ingredients:

- 1/2 cup cooked quinoa
- 1/4 cup almond milk
- 1/2 cup mixed berries (such as strawberries, blueberries, raspberries)
- 1 tablespoon chopped nuts (such as almonds, walnuts)
- 1 tablespoon honey or maple syrup (optional)

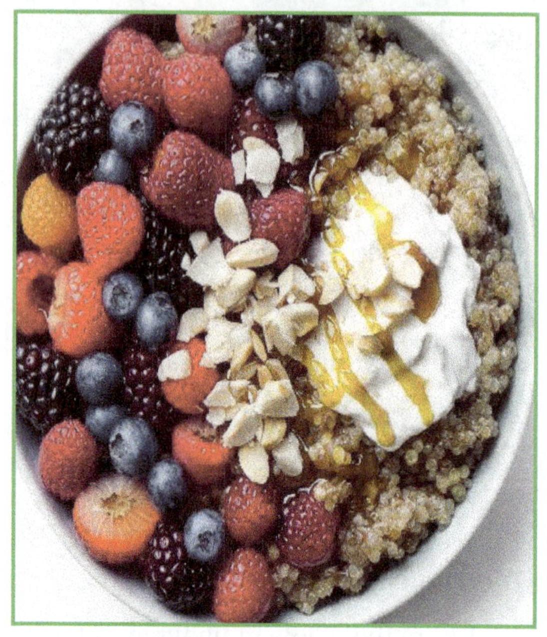

Directions:

1. In a bowl, combine cooked quinoa and almond milk. Stir well.
2. Top with mixed berries, chopped nuts, and a drizzle of honey or maple syrup if desired.
3. Serve warm or chilled.

Nutritional information:

Calories: 280

Protein: 7g

Carbohydrates: 45g

Fiber: 7g

Fat: 9g

Ingredients:

- 6 eggs
- 1 cup chopped spinach
- 1/2 cup sliced mushrooms
- 1/4 cup diced onions
- Salt and pepper to taste
- Use cooking spray or olive oil for greasing.

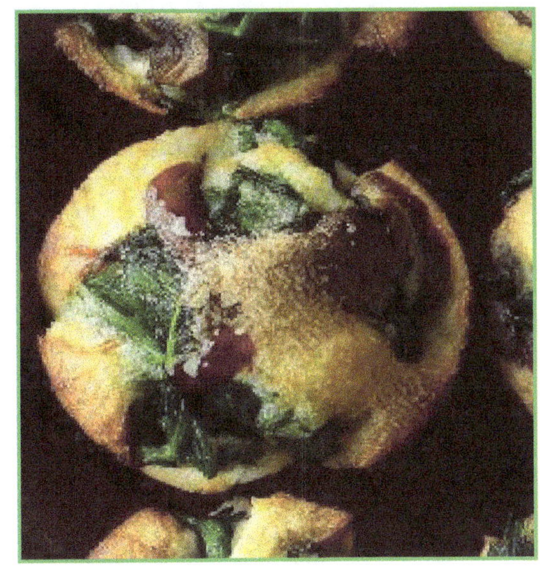

Directions:

1. Preheat oven to 350°F (175°C). Coat a muffin tray with a cooking spray or olive oil.
2. In a mixing bowl, stir the eggs, salt, and pepper.
3. Stir in chopped spinach, sliced mushrooms, and diced onions.
4. Pour the egg mixture equally across the prepared muffin tray.
5. Bake for 15-20 minutes or until the egg muffins are set and lightly golden on top.
6. Allow to cool slightly before removing from the muffin tin.
7. Serve warm or store in the refrigerator for later use.

Nutritional information:

Calories: 180

Protein: 14g

Carbohydrates: 3g

Fiber: 1g

Fat: 12g

Ingredients:

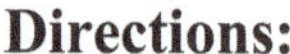

- 1/2 cup low-fat cottage cheese
- 1/2 cup mixed fresh fruits (such as diced apples, berries, bananas)
- 1 tablespoon chopped nuts or seeds (such as almonds, pumpkin seeds)
- 1 teaspoon of honey (optional)

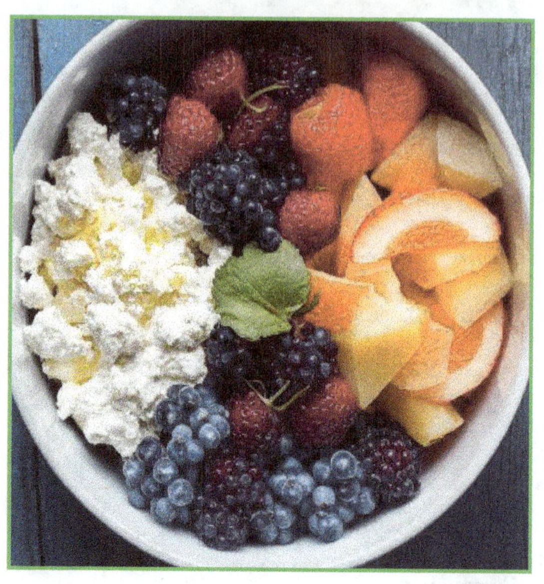

Directions:

1. Spoon low-fat cottage cheese into a bowl.
2. Top with mixed fresh fruits and chopped nuts or seeds.
3. Sprinkle either with honey as desired.
4. Serve chilled.

Nutritional information:

Calories: 220

Protein: 18g

Carbohydrates: 20g

Fiber: 3g

Fat: 8g

Ingredients:

- 1 small sweet potato that has been peeled and chopped
- 1/2 onion, diced
- 1 bell pepper, diced
- 2 eggs
- Salt, pepper, and paprika to taste
- Cooking oil (such as olive oil or coconut oil)

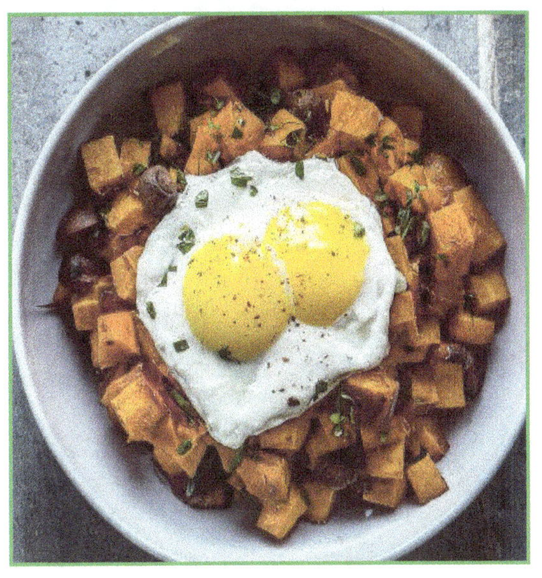

Directions:

1. Heat cooking oil in a skillet over medium heat.
2. Add diced sweet potato, onion, and bell pepper to the skillet.
3. Season with salt, pepper, and paprika.
4. Cook, stirring occasionally, until sweet potatoes are tender and slightly crispy on the edges.
5. Create two wells in the hash mixture and crack an egg into each well.
6. Cover the skillet and cook until the eggs are cooked to your liking (runny or firm).
7. Serve hot, optionally garnished with fresh herbs.

Nutritional information:

Calories: 320

Protein: 15g

Carbohydrates: 30g

Fiber: 5g

Fat: 15g

Ingredients:

- 1 cup of cauliflower rice
- 1/2 cup of cooked black beans
- 1/4 avocado, sliced
- 2 tablespoons of salsa
- 1 tablespoon chopped cilantro
- 1 lime, cut into wedges

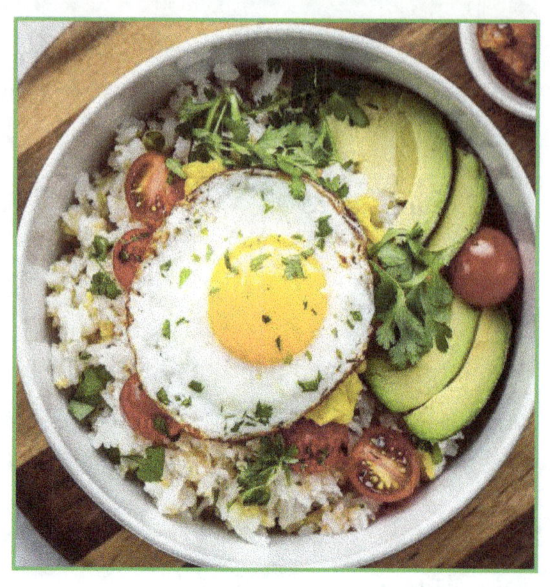

Directions:

1. In a skillet, heat cauliflower rice and cooked black beans until warmed through.
2. Spoon the cauliflower rice and black beans into a bowl.
3. Top with sliced avocado, salsa, chopped cilantro, and a squeeze of lime juice.
4. Mix everything together and enjoy.

Nutritional information:

Calories: 280

Protein: 12g

Carbohydrates: 30g

Fiber: 12g

Fat: 14g

Ingredients:

- 1 whole grain tortilla
- 2 eggs, scrambled
- 1/4 cup of sliced bell peppers, any color
- 1/4 cup diced tomatoes
- Fresh spinach leaves
- Add spices such as pepper, salt, and cumin to taste.
- Salsa or hot sauce (optional)

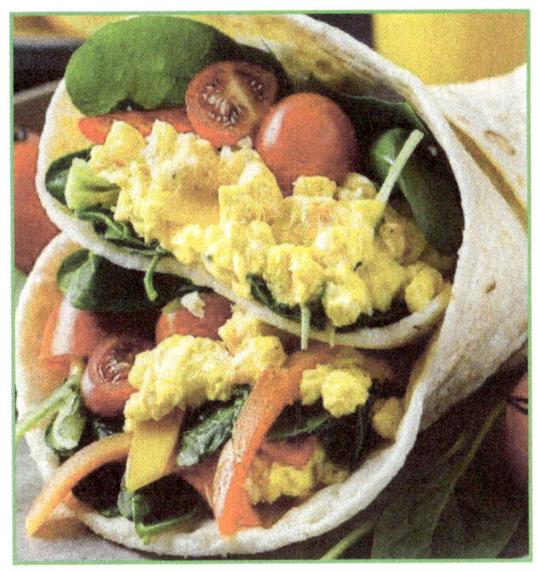

Directions:

1. Warm the whole grain wrap or tortilla in a skillet or microwave.
2. Layer scrambled eggs, diced bell peppers, diced tomatoes, fresh spinach leaves, and season with salt, pepper, and cumin.
3. Add salsa or hot sauce if desired.
4. Roll up the wrap tightly, cut in half if desired, and serve.

Nutritional information:

Calories: 280

Protein: 15g

Carbohydrates: 25g

Fiber: 8g

Fat: 12g

Ingredients:

- 1 cup of Greek yogurt
- 1/2 cup mixed berries (such as strawberries, blueberries, raspberries)
- 2 tablespoons granola
- 1 tablespoon honey or maple syrup (optional)

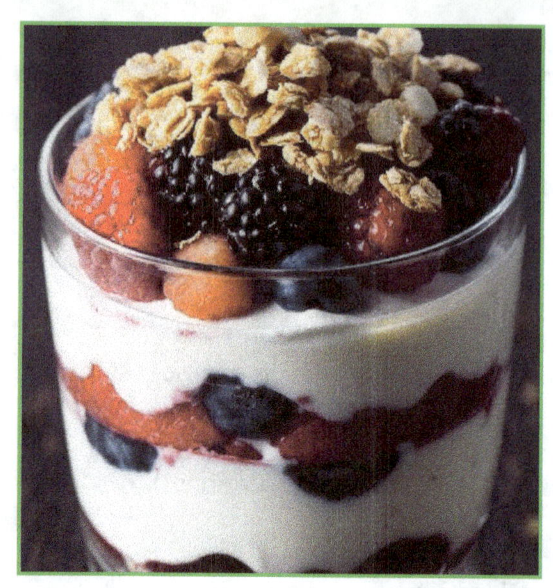

Directions:

1. In a glass or bowl, layer Greek yogurt, mixed berries, and granola.
2. Drizzle with honey or maple syrup if desired.
3. Repeat the layers until all ingredients are used.
4. Serve chilled.

Nutritional information:

Calories: 280

Protein: 20g

Carbohydrates: 35g

Fiber: 6g

Fat: 7g

Ingredients:

- 2 eggs
- 1/4 cup chopped spinach
- 2 tablespoons shredded cheddar cheese
- Salt and pepper to taste
- 1 teaspoon olive oil or butter

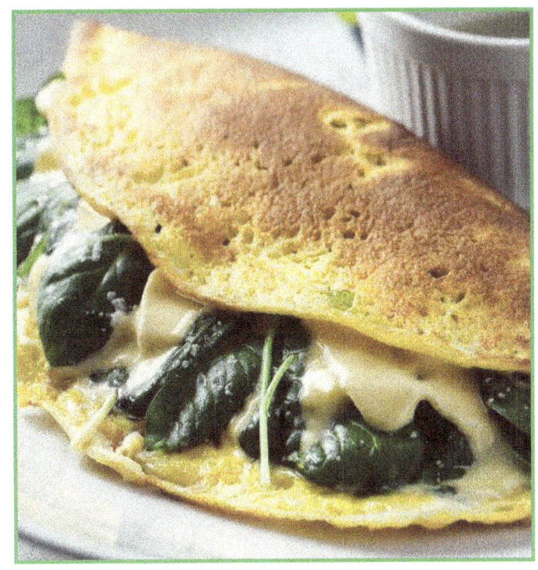

Directions:

1. In a mixing bowl, batter the eggs, salt, and pepper.
2. Heat olive oil or butter in a non-stick skillet over medium heat.
3. Pour the batter egg into the skillet.
4. Sprinkle chopped spinach and shredded cheddar cheese evenly over the eggs.
5. Cook until the eggs are set and the cheese is melted.
6. Fold the omelette in halves and place on a plate.
7. Serve hot.

Nutritional information:

Calories: 280

Protein: 18g

Carbohydrates: 2g

Fiber: 1g

Fat: 21g

Ingredients:

- 1/2 cup mixed berries (such as strawberries, blueberries, raspberries)
- 1 tablespoon chia seeds
- 1/2 cup almond milk
- 1/2 cup Greek yogurt
- 1 teaspoon honey or maple syrup (optional)

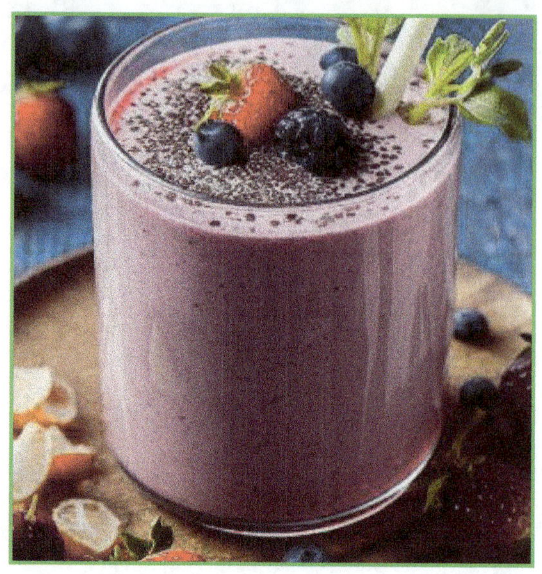

Directions:

1. In a blender, combine mixed berries, chia seeds, almond milk, Greek yogurt, and honey or maple syrup.
2. Blend until smooth and creamy.
3. Pour into a glass and serve immediately.

Nutritional information:

Calories: 220

Protein: 10g

Carbohydrates: 25g

Fiber: 8g

Fat: 9g

Ingredients:

- 1/2 cup almond flour
- 2 eggs
- 1/4 cup almond milk
- 1/2 teaspoon baking powder
- 1 tablespoon coconut oil (for cooking)
- Fresh berries for topping (optional)
- Maple syrup or honey (optional)

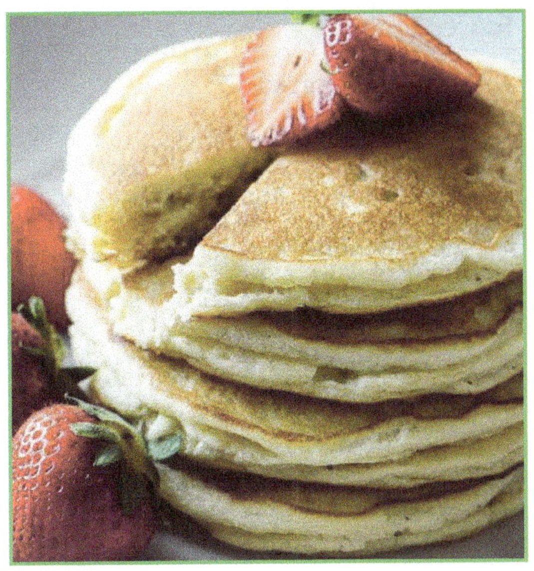

Directions:

1. In a bowl, whisk together almond flour, eggs, almond milk, and baking powder until smooth.
2. Heat coconut oil in a non-stick skillet over medium heat.
3. Pour batter onto the skillet to form small pancakes.
4. Cook until bubbles form on the surface, then flip and cook until golden brown on both sides.
5. Serve pancakes topped with fresh berries and a drizzle of maple syrup or honey if desired.

Nutritional information:

Calories: 280

Protein: 12g

Carbohydrates: 10g

Fiber: 4g

Fat: 20g

Ingredients:

- 1/2 avocado, diced
- 2 eggs, boiled or poached
- 1/2 cup cooked quinoa or brown rice
- 1/4 cup cherry tomatoes, halved
- Salt and pepper to taste
- Fresh cilantro or parsley for garnish

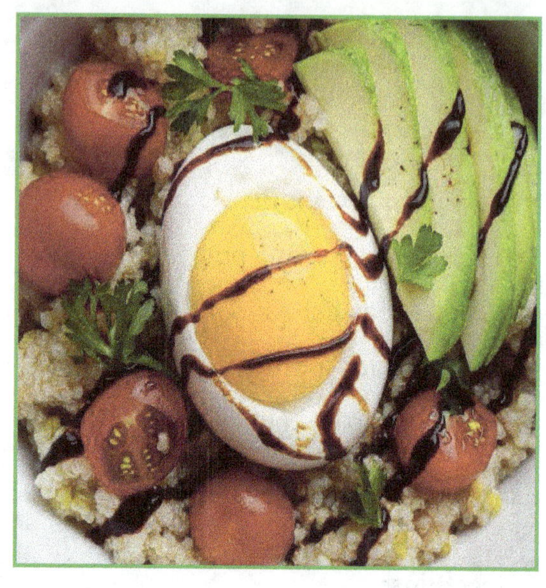

Directions:

1. In a bowl, combine diced avocado, boiled or poached eggs, cooked quinoa or brown rice, and halved cherry tomatoes.
2. Season with salt and pepper.
3. Garnish with freshly chopped parsley or cilantro.
4. Serve warm or chilled.

Nutritional information:

Calories: 320

Protein: 15g

Carbohydrates: 20g

Fiber: 8g

Fat: 22g

Ingredients:

- 2 tablespoons of chia seeds
- 1/2 cup of coconut milk
- 1/2 cup diced mango
- 1 tablespoon shredded coconut
- 1 teaspoon honey or maple syrup (optional)

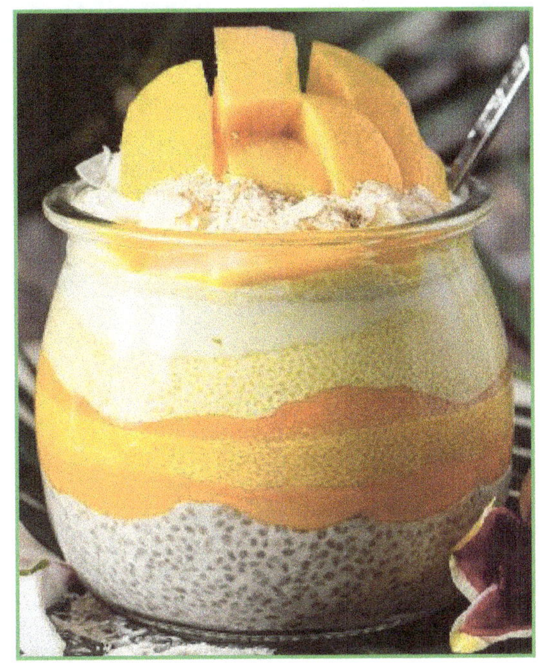

Directions:

1. In a bowl, stir the chia seeds and coconut milk together. Let it sit for 10 minutes.
2. Stir the mixture again to prevent clumping.
3. Layer diced mango at the bottom of a glass or jar.
4. Pour the chia seed mixture over the mango.
5. Top with shredded coconut and drizzle with honey or maple syrup if desired.
6. Refrigerate for minimum of two hours, or overnight.
7. Serve chilled.

Nutritional information:

Calories: 280

Protein: 5g

Carbohydrates: 30g

Fiber: 8g

Fat: 18g

Ingredients:

- 4 egg whites
- 1/2 cup diced bell peppers (any color)
- 1/4 cup diced onions
- 1/4 cup diced tomatoes
- Pepper and salt to enrich the taste
- 1 teaspoon olive oil

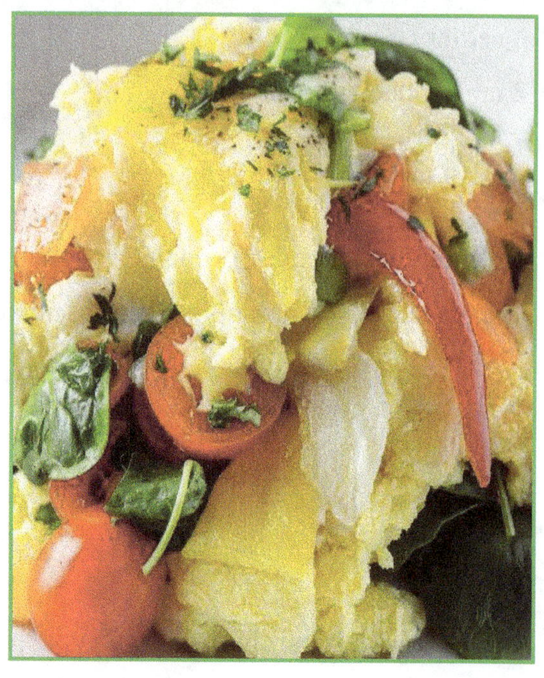

Directions:

1. With medium heat, heat the olive oil in a skillet.
2. Add diced onions and bell peppers to the skillet. Sauté until softened.
3. Pour in egg whites and stir gently.
4. Add diced tomatoes and continue cooking until the eggs are cooked through.
5. Season with salt and pepper.
6. Serve hot.

Nutritional information:

Calories: 120

Protein: 15g

Carbohydrates: 8g

Fiber: 2g

Fat: 4g

Ingredients:

- 2 tablespoons chia seeds
- 1/2 cup almond milk (or any milk of choice)
- 1/2 teaspoon vanilla extract
- Fresh fruit for topping (such as sliced strawberries, kiwi, or mango)
- 1 tablespoon chopped nuts (optional)

Directions:

1. In a bowl, combine chia seeds, almond milk, and vanilla extract. Stir well.
2. Let the mixture sit for about 10 minutes, stirring occasionally until it thickens.
3. Transfer the chia seed pudding into a serving bowl.
4. Top with fresh fruit and chopped nuts.
5. Serve chilled.

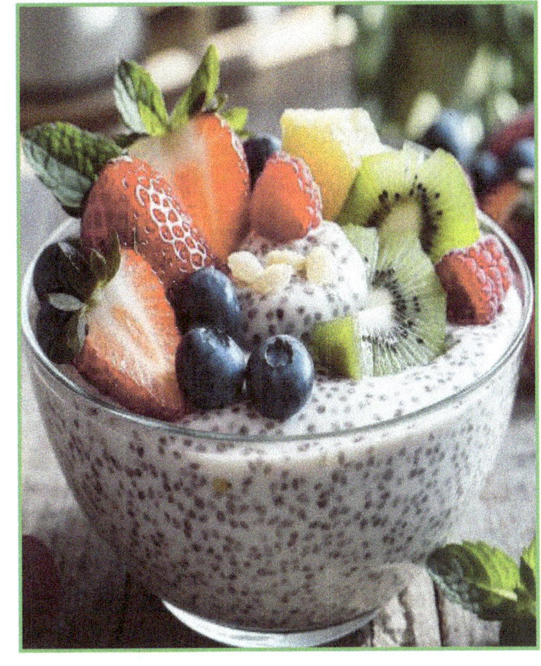

Nutritional information:

Calories: 220

Protein: 5g

Carbohydrates: 25g

Fiber: 10g

Fat: 12g

Ingredients:

- 1 ripe mango, scraped and slice
- 1/2 cup coconut milk
- 1/2 cup Greek yogurt
- 1 tablespoon honey or agave syrup (optional)
- Ice cubes

Directions:

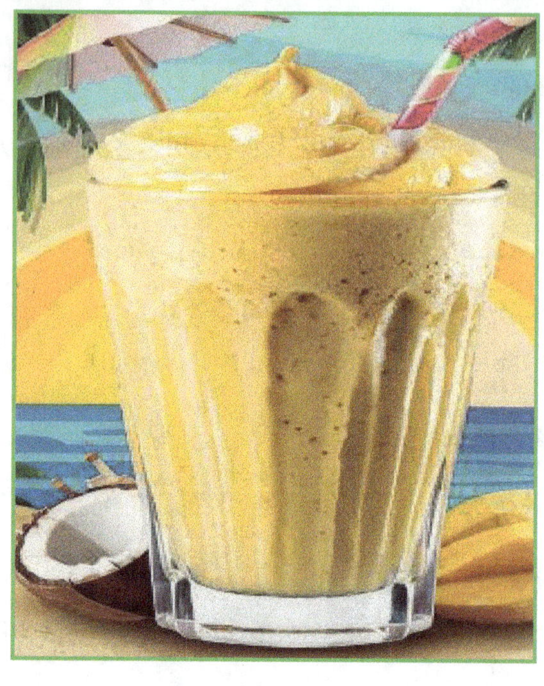

Nutritional information:

Calories: 280

Protein: 8g

Carbohydrates: 35g

Fiber: 4g

Fat: 14g

Ingredients:

- 2 hard-boiled eggs, sliced
- 1/2 avocado, sliced
- 1 cup mixed greens (such as spinach, arugula, or kale)
- Cherry tomatoes, halved
- 1 tablespoon olive oil
- 1 tablespoon balsamic vinegar
- Pepper and salt to enrich the taste
-

Directions:

1. In a bowl, toss mixed greens and cherry tomatoes with olive oil, balsamic vinegar, salt, and pepper.
2. Arrange the sliced hard-boiled eggs and avocado on top of the salad.
3. Serve immediately as a refreshing breakfast salad.

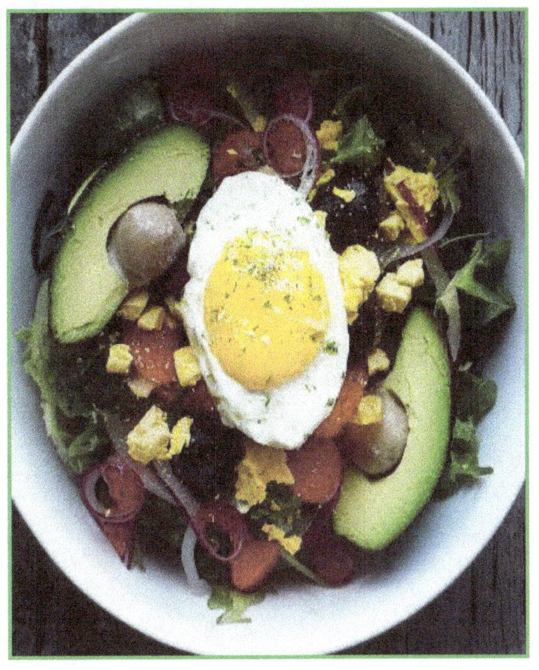

Nutritional information:

Calories: 320

Protein: 12g

Carbohydrates: 10g

Fiber: 6g

Fat: 25g

PHASE 2
LOW RESIDUAL DIET (FOR RECOVERY)

CHAPTER 5

LOW RESIDUAL DIET (FOR RECOVERY) RECIPES

GRILLED CHICKEN SALAD WITH AVOCADO

Ingredients:

- 4 oz grilled chicken breast, sliced
- 2 cups of mixed greens (the spinach, arugula, and lettuce)
- 1/2 avocado, sliced
- 1/4 cup cherry tomatoes, halved
- 1/4 cup cucumber, sliced
- 1 tablespoon olive oil
- 1 tablespoon balsamic vinegar
- - Salt and

Directions:

1. In a large bowl, combine mixed greens, cherry tomatoes, cucumber, and avocado slices.
2. Add sliced grilled chicken on top.
3. Sprinkle with olive oil and balsamic vinegar to taste. Season with salt and pepper.
4. Toss gently to coat everything evenly.
5. Serve immediately.

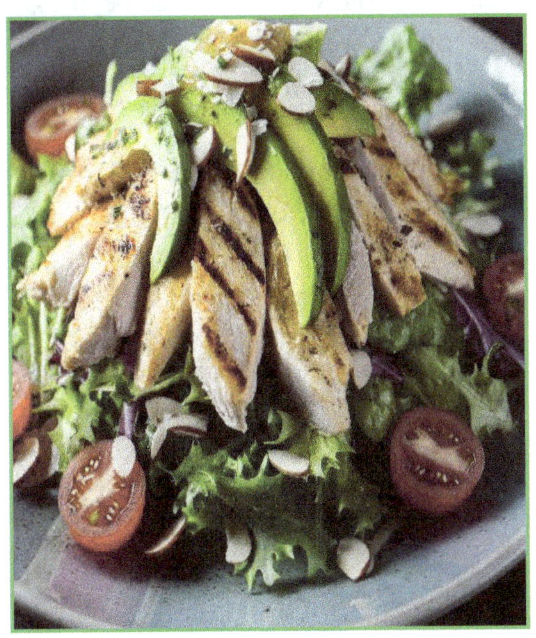

Nutritional information:

Calories: 320

Protein: 30g

Carbohydrates: 10g

Fiber: 6g

Fat: 18g

Ingredients:

- 1/2 cup quinoa, cooked
- 1 cup of mixed vegetables (red peppers, broccoli, and carrots)
- 1/4 cup diced onion
- 2 cloves garlic, minced
- 2 tablespoons soy sauce (low-sodium)
- 1 tablespoon olive oil
- Salt and pepper to taste
- Sliced tofu or chicken for added protein (optional)

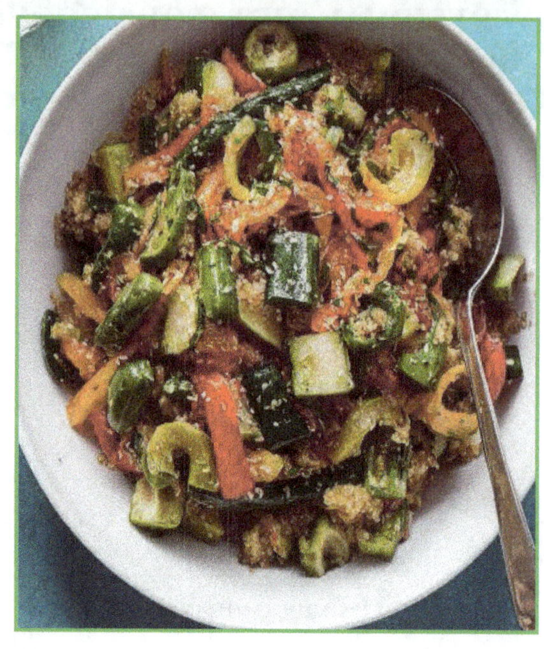

Directions:

1. In a medium-sized pan, heat the olive oil.
2. Sauté diced onion and minced garlic until tasty.
3. Add mixed vegetables and cook until tender-crisp.
4. Stir in cooked quinoa and soy sauce.
5. Season with salt and pepper to taste.
6. Optionally, add sliced tofu or chicken and cook until heated through.
7. Serve hot.

Nutritional information:

Calories: 280

Protein: 12g

Carbohydrates: 40g

Fiber: 8g

Fat: 8g

Ingredients:

- 6 oz salmon fillet
- 1 cup asparagus spears
- 1/2 lemon, sliced
- 1 tablespoon olive oil
- Fresh dill (optional)
- Salt and pepper to taste

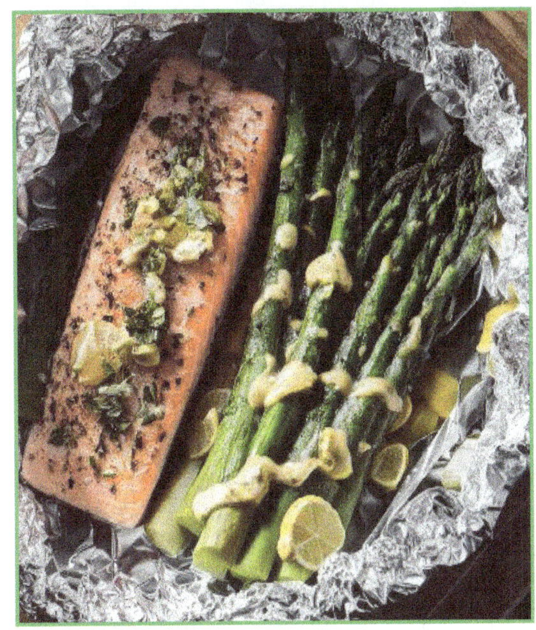

Directions:

1. Preheat oven to 400°F (200°C).
2. Place salmon fillet on a piece of aluminum foil.
3. Arrange asparagus spears around the salmon.
4. Drizzle olive oil over the salmon and asparagus.
5. Season with salt, pepper, and fresh dill.
6. Place lemon slices on top of the salmon.
7. Fold the aluminum foil to create a sealed packet.
8. Bake in the preheated oven for 15-20 minutes or until salmon is cooked through.
9. Carefully open the foil packet and serve hot.

Nutritional information:

Calories: 320

Protein: 30g

Carbohydrates: 8g

Fiber: 4g

Fat: 18g

Ingredients:

- 8 oz ground turkey
- 4 cups low-sodium chicken broth
- 1 cup diced carrots
- 1 cup diced celery
- 1 cup diced zucchini
- 1/2 cup diced onion
- 2 cloves garlic, minced
- 1 teaspoon dried thyme
- Salt and pepper to taste
- Fresh parsley for garnish

Directions:

1. In a pot, brown ground turkey over medium heat.
2. Sauté diced onion and minced garlic until translucent.
3. Pour in the chicken broth then bring it to a boil.
4. Add diced carrots, celery, zucchini, and dried thyme.
5. Season with salt and pepper to taste.
6. Simmer for about 15-20 minutes until vegetables are tender.
7. Serve hot, garnished with fresh parsley.

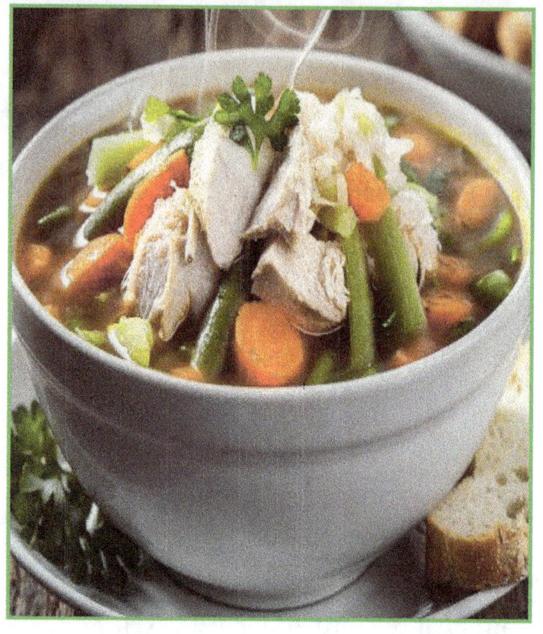

Nutritional information:

Calories: 280

Protein: 25g

Carbohydrates: 15g

Fiber: 4g

Fat: 12g

Ingredients:
- 1 can (15 oz) of chickpeas, rinsed and drained
- 1 cup cherry tomatoes, halved
- 1/2 cucumber, diced
- 1/4 cup red onion, finely chopped
- 1/4 cup chopped fresh parsley
- 2 tablespoons olive oil
- 1 tablespoon lemon juice
- 1 teaspoon dried oregano
- Salt and pepper to taste
- Feta cheese (optional)

Directions:
1. In a large bowl, combine chickpeas, cherry tomatoes, cucumber, red onion, and fresh parsley.
2. In a small bowl, mix the olive oil, lemon juice, the dried oregano, salt, and pepper.
3. Dump the dressing on the salad and mix to coat evenly.
4. If desired, crumble feta cheese on top before serving.
5. Serve chilled or at ambient temperature.

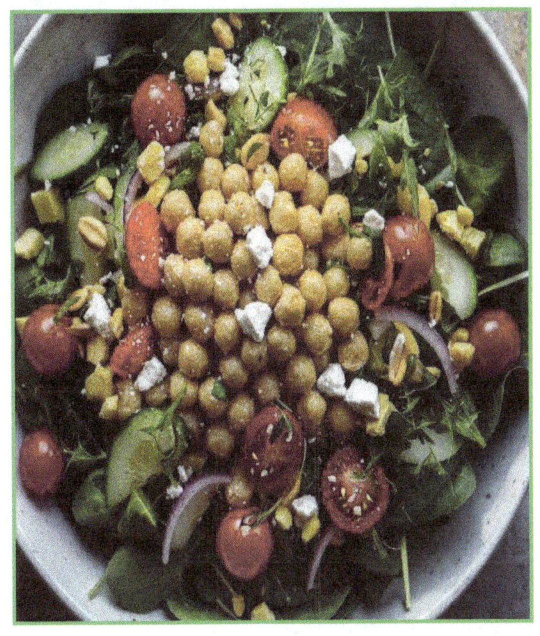

Nutritional information:

Calories: 280

Protein: 10g

Carbohydrates: 30g

Fiber: 8g

Fat: 14g

Ingredients:

- 2 bell peppers, halved and seeded
- 1 small eggplant, diced
- 1 cup marinara sauce (low-sodium)
- 1 cup shredded mozzarella cheese
- 2 tablespoons grated Parmesan cheese
- Fresh basil leaves for garnish
- Olive oil for cooking
- Salt and pepper to taste

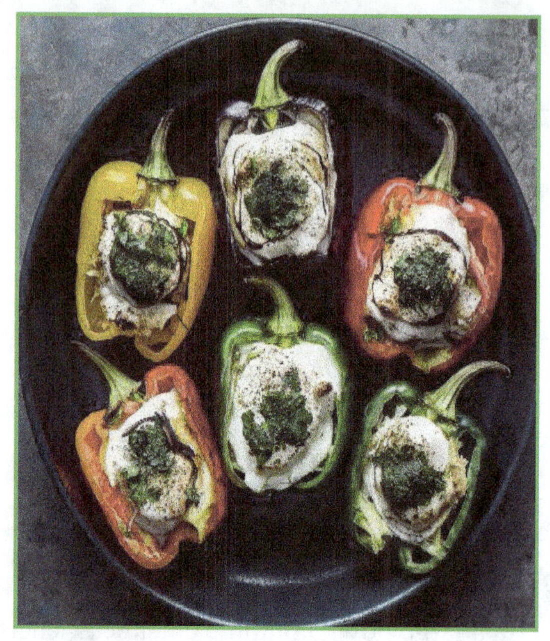

Directions:

1. Preheat oven to 375°F (190°C).
2. In a medium-sized pan, heat the olive oil.
3. Add diced eggplant and sauté until softened.
4. Season with salt and pepper.
5. Stir in marinara sauce and simmer for a few minutes.
6. Fill each halved bell pepper with the eggplant mixture.
7. Top with shredded mozzarella and grated Parmesan cheese.
8. Place stuffed bell peppers on a baking dish and cover with foil.
9. Bake in the preheated oven for 25-30 minutes or until the peppers are tender and the cheese is melted and bubbly.
10. Remove from the oven to allow it cool slightly.
11. Toss with fresh basil leaves while serving.

Nutritional information:

Calories: 220

Protein: 10g

Carbohydrates: 20g

Fiber: 6g

Fat: 12g

Ingredients:

- 1 cup dried lentils, rinsed
- 4 cups low-sodium vegetable broth
- 1 cup diced carrots
- 1 cup diced celery
- 1 cup diced potatoes
- 1/2 cup diced onion
- 2 cloves garlic, minced
- 1 teaspoon ground cumin
- 1 teaspoon paprika
- Salt and pepper to enrich the taste
- Fresh parsley for garnish

Directions:

1. In a pot, combine dried lentils, vegetable broth, diced carrots, celery, potatoes, onion, and garlic.
2. Add ground cumin, paprika, salt, and pepper.
3. Bring to a boil, then reduce heat and simmer uncovered for about 25-30 minutes or until lentils and vegetables are tender.
4. Adjust seasoning if needed.
5. Serve hot and drizzled with fresh parsley.

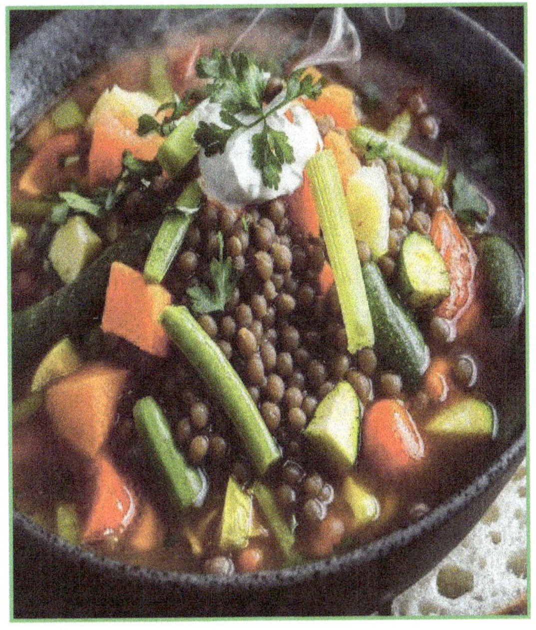

Nutritional information:

Calories: 280

Protein: 15g

Carbohydrates: 45g

Fiber: 12g

Fat: 2g

Ingredients:

- 8 ounces of shrimp, peeled and deveined
- 2 small zucchinis, spiralized into pasta.
- 1 bell pepper, sliced
- 1/4 cup sliced mushrooms
- 2 tablespoons low-sodium soy sauce
- 1 tablespoon olive oil
- 1 teaspoon minced ginger
- 2 cloves garlic, minced
- Salt and pepper to taste
- Sesame seeds for garnish

Directions:

1. Heat the olive oil with a medium heat in pan.
2. Add minced ginger and garlic, sauté until fragrant.
3. Add shrimp to the pan and cook until pink and cooked through. Take the prawn from the pan and put aside.
4. In the same pan, add sliced bell pepper and mushrooms. Cook until tender.
5. Add zucchini noodles and soy sauce to the pan. Cook for a few minutes until noodles are just tender.
6. Return the cooked shrimp to the pan and toss everything together.
7. Mix little salt and pepper to taste.
8. Sprinkle with fresh sesame seeds prior to serving.

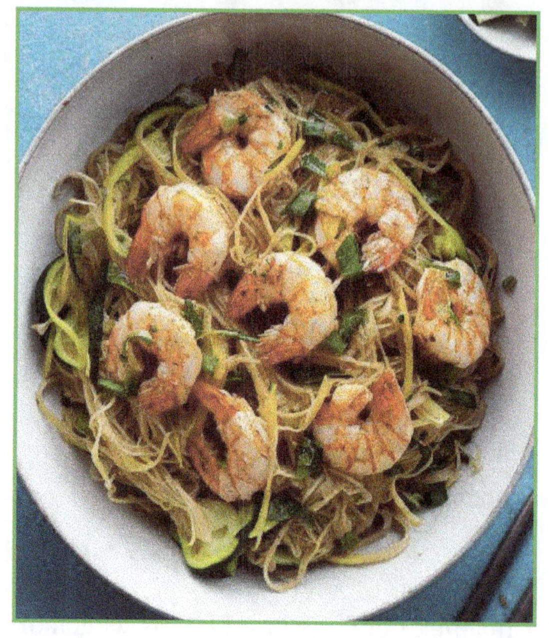

Nutritional information:

Calories: 280

Protein: 25g

Carbohydrates: 15g

Fiber: 5g

Fat: 12g

Ingredients:

- 8 oz chicken breast, cut into cubes
- 1 bell pepper, cut into chunks
- 1 zucchini, sliced
- 1 red onion sliced into quarters.
- 1 tablespoon olive oil
- 1 teaspoon of dried herbs like thyme and rosemary leaves
- Salt and pepper to taste
- Wooden or metal skewers

Directions:

1. Prepare the grill pan by preheating it on medium-high heat.
2. Thread chicken cubes, bell pepper chunks, zucchini slices, and onion wedges onto skewers.
3. Brush skewers with olive oil and sprinkle with dried herbs, salt, and pepper.
4. Grill the skewers for 10-12 minutes, flipping regularly, until the chicken is fully cooked and the veggies become charred and soft.
5. Remove from the grill and allow it cool for a few minutes' prior serving.

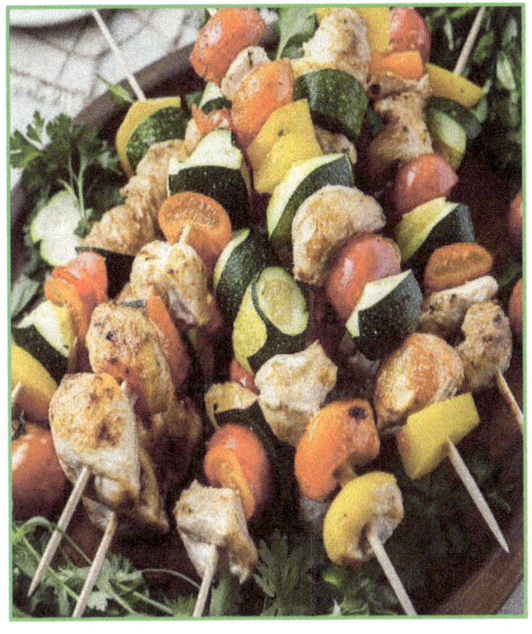

Nutritional information:

Calories: 280

Protein: 30g

Carbohydrates: 10g

Fiber: 3g

Fat: 12g

Ingredients:

- 1 medium spaghetti squash
- 2 cups tomato basil sauce (low-sodium)
- 1/4 cup grated Parmesan cheese
- Fresh basil leaves for garnish
- Olive oil for drizzling
- Salt and pepper to enrich taste

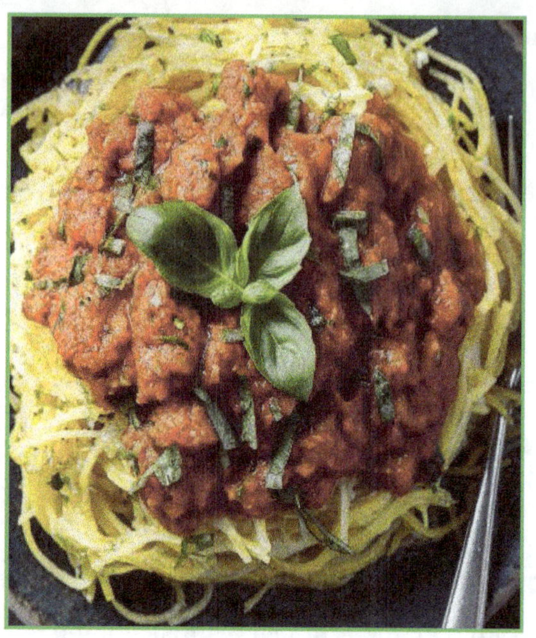

Directions:

1. Preheat oven to 400°F (200°C)
2. Split the spaghetti squash in halves lengthwise, then scrape out the seeds.
3. Pour olive oil over the squash's sliced sides and season with salt and pepper.
4. Lay the squash in halves, cut side down over a baking sheet lined with parchment paper.
5. Roast in the preheated oven for about 30-40 minutes or until the squash is tender and the flesh can be easily shredded with a fork.
6. Transfer from the oven and wait for it to cool slightly.
7. Use a fork to scrape the squash flesh into strands (like spaghetti) and transfer to a bowl.
8. Heat tomato basil sauce in a saucepan until warmed through.
9. Pour the sauce over the spaghetti squash and toss to coat evenly.
10. Sprinkle grated Parmesan cheese and garnish with fresh basil leaves before serving

Nutritional information:

Calories: 220

Protein: 5g

Carbohydrates: 35g

Fiber: 8g

Fat: 8g

Ingredients:

- 4 oz grilled chicken breast, sliced
- 2 cups mixed greens (romaine lettuce, cucumber, red onion, olives)
- 1/4 cup crumbled feta cheese
- 1/4 cup cherry tomatoes, halved
- 1/4 cup sliced cucumbers
- 1/4 cup sliced red onion
- 2 tablespoons Greek dressing (low-fat)
- Fresh oregano for garnish
- Salt and pepper to taste

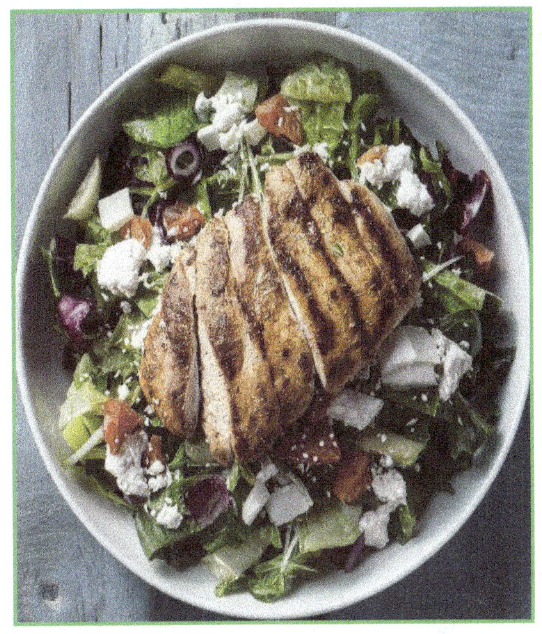

Directions:

1. In a large bowl, combine mixed greens, cherry tomatoes, sliced cucumbers, and red onion.
2. Add grilled chicken slices on top.
3. Sprinkle crumbled feta cheese over the salad.
4. Drizzle Greek dressing and toss gently to coat everything.
5. Season with salt, pepper, and garnish with fresh oregano.
6. Serve immediately.

Nutritional information:

Calories: 320

Protein: 30g

Carbohydrates: 10g

Fiber: 4g

Fat: 18g

Ingredients:

- 1/2 cup quinoa, cooked
- 1/2 cup black beans, cooked
- 1/4 cup corn kernels (fresh or canned)
- 1/4 cup sliced bell peppers
- 1/4 cup diced tomatoes
- 2 tablespoons chopped cilantro
- 1 tablespoon lime juice
- 1 tablespoon olive oil
- Salt and pepper to taste
- Avocado slices for garnish

Directions:

1. In a bowl, combine cooked quinoa, black beans, corn kernels, diced bell peppers, diced tomatoes, chopped cilantro, lime juice, olive oil, salt, and pepper.
2. Toss everything until thoroughly blended.
3. Transfer the quinoa and black bean mixture into a serving bowl.
4. Garnish with avocado slices on top.
5. Serve at ambient temperature or chilled.

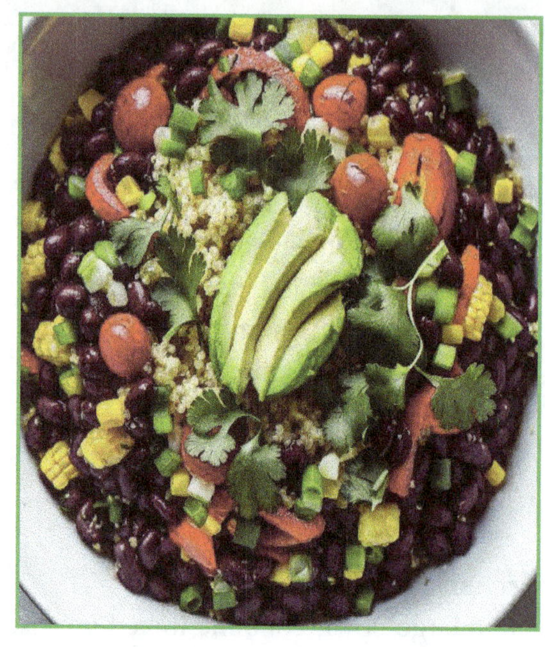

Nutritional information:

Calories: 280

Protein: 10g

Carbohydrates: 35g

Fiber: 8g

Fat: 12g

Ingredients:

- 8 oz ground turkey
- 2 cups of mixed veggies (broccoli, bell peppers, snap peas).
- 2 cloves garlic, minced
- 2 tablespoons low-sodium soy sauce
- 1 tablespoon olive oil
- 1 teaspoon grated ginger
- Salt and pepper to taste
- Cooked brown rice for serving

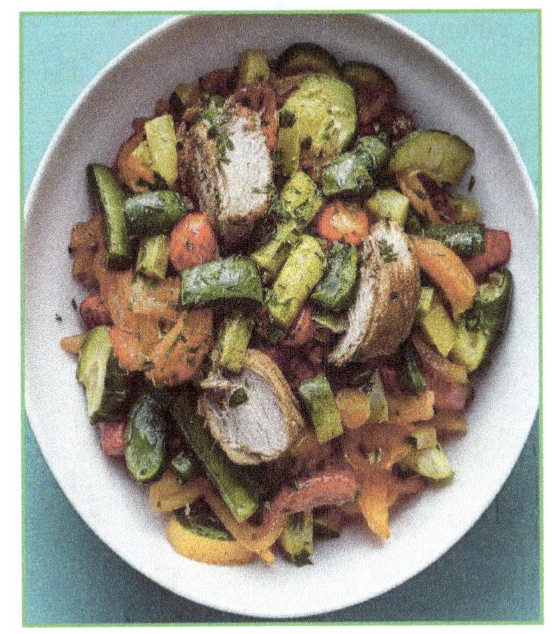

Directions:

1. Heat the olive oil in a skillet or wok over medium-high heat.
2. Add minced garlic and grated ginger, sauté until fragrant.
3. Cook the ground turkey in a pan until it's browned.
4. Add mixed vegetables and stir-fry for a few minutes until vegetables are tender-crisp.
5. Pour in soy sauce and toss everything together.
6. Garnish with pepper and salt to taste.
7. Serve the turkey and vegetable stir-fry over cooked brown rice.

Nutritional information:

Calories: 320

Protein: 25g

Carbohydrates: 30g

Fiber: 6g

Fat: 12g

Ingredients:

- 1 can (15 ounce) of chickpeas, rinsed and drained
- 1/2 cup diced cucumber
- 1/2 cup diced tomatoes
- 1/4 cup diced red onion
- 2 tablespoons chopped fresh parsley
- 2 tablespoons olive oil
- 1 tablespoon lemon juice
- 1 teaspoon dried oregano
- Salt and pepper to taste
- Whole grain wraps or tortillas
- Optional: crumbled feta cheese, hummus

Directions:

1. In a bowl, combine chickpeas, diced cucumber, diced tomatoes, diced red onion, chopped parsley, olive oil, lemon juice, dried oregano, salt, and pepper.

2. Toss everything until thoroughly blended.

3. Warm the whole grain wraps or tortillas.

4. Spread hummus (if using) on the wraps.

5. Spoon the chickpea mixture onto the wraps.

6. Optionally, sprinkle with crumbled feta cheese.

7. Roll up the wraps tightly and serve.

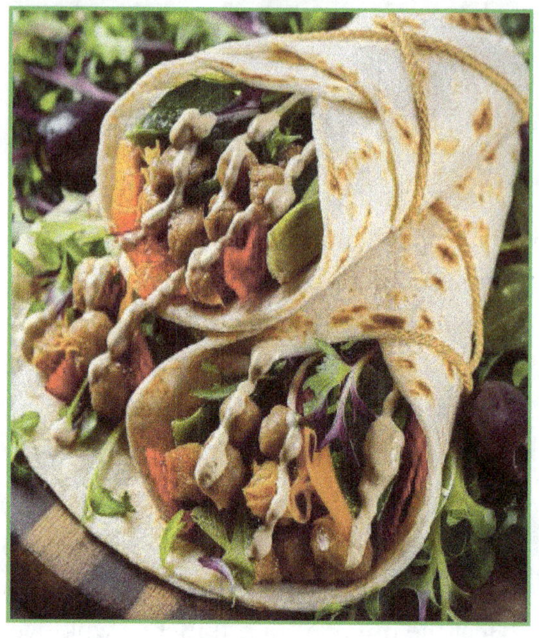

Nutritional information:

Calories: 280

Protein: 10g

Carbohydrates: 35g

Fiber: 8g

Fat: 12g

Ingredients:

- 4 boneless, skinless chicken breasts
- 1 cup chopped spinach
- 1/2 cup sliced mushrooms
- 1/4 cup diced onion
- 2 cloves garlic, minced
- 1/4 cup shredded mozzarella cheese
- 1 tablespoon olive oil
- Salt and pepper to taste
- Toothpicks or kitchen twine

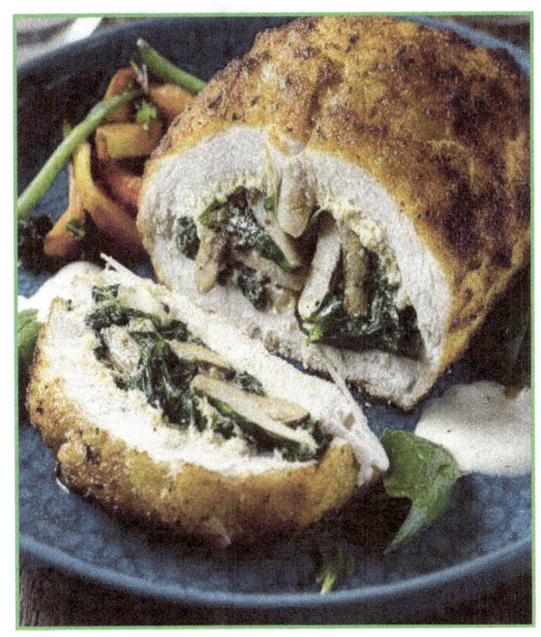

Directions:

1. Preheat oven to 375°F (190°C).
2. In a saucepan, heat the olive oil on a low flame.
3. Add diced onion and minced garlic, sauté until softened.
4. Stir in chopped spinach and sliced mushrooms, cook until vegetables are tender and moisture has evaporated.
5. Season with salt and pepper.
6. Butterfly each chicken breast by slicing horizontally through the middle, but not cutting all the way through.
7. Stuff each chicken breast with the spinach and mushroom mixture.
8. Sprinkle shredded mozzarella cheese over the stuffing.
9. Secure the chicken breasts with toothpicks or tie with kitchen twine.
10. Place stuffed chicken breasts on a baking sheet and bake in the preheated oven for 25-30 minutes or until chicken is cooked through and juices run clear.
11. Remove toothpicks or twine before serving.

Nutritional information:

Calories: 320

Protein: 30g

Carbohydrates: 5g

Fiber: 2g

Fat: 18g

Ingredients:

- 4 big bell peppers, half & seeds removed
- 1 cup quinoa, cooked
- 1 can (15 oz) black beans, drained and rinsed
- 1 cup corn kernels (fresh or frozen)
- 1/2 cup diced tomatoes
- 1/2 cup shredded cheddar cheese
- 1 teaspoon chili powder
- 1/2 teaspoon cumin
- Salt and pepper to taste
- Fresh cilantro for garnish

Directions:

1. Preheat oven to 375°F (190°C).
2. 2. In a large bowl, combine cooked quinoa, black beans, corn kernels, diced tomatoes, shredded cheddar cheese, chili powder, cumin, salt, and pepper.
3. Mix everything until well combined.
4. Fill each halved bell pepper with the quinoa and vegetable mixture.
5. Place stuffed peppers in a baking dish and cover with foil.
6. Bake in a preheated oven for approximately 25-30 minutes.
7. Remove the foil and sprinkle extra cheese on top of each stuffed pepper if desired.
8. Bake uncovered for an additional 5 minutes or until cheese is melted and bubbly.
9. Garnish with fresh cilantro before serving.

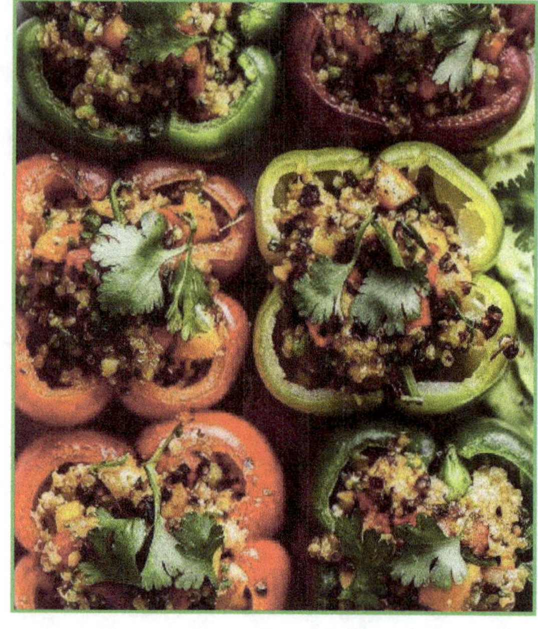

Nutritional information:

Calories: 320

Protein: 15g

Carbohydrates: 45g

Fiber: 12g

Fat: 10g

Ingredients:

- 1 can of 5-ounce tuna in water, drained
- 1/4 cup diced celery
- 1/4 cup diced red onion
- 2 tablespoons chopped pickles
- 2 tablespoons plain Greek yogurt
- 1 tablespoon Dijon mustard
- 1 tablespoon lemon juice
- Salt and pepper to taste
- Lettuce leaves for wrapping (such as Romaine or Butter lettuce)
- Sliced avocado (optional)

Directions:

1. In a bowl, combine drained tuna, diced celery, diced red onion, chopped pickles, Greek yogurt, Dijon mustard, lemon juice, salt, and pepper.

2. Mix until well combined.

3. Spoon the tuna salad mixture onto lettuce leaves.

4. Add sliced avocado on top if desired.

5. Roll up the lettuce leaves to form wraps.

6. Serve immediately.

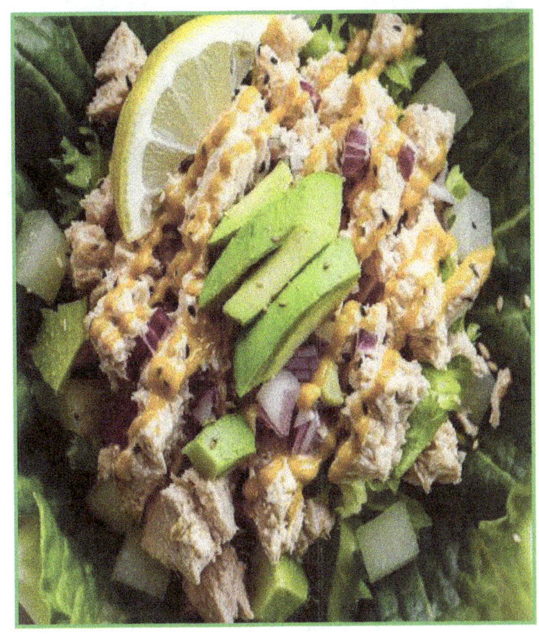

Nutritional information:

Calories: 220

Protein: 25g

Carbohydrates: 10g

Fiber: 4g

Fat: 8g

Ingredients:

- 2 small zucchinis, spiralized into pasta.
- 1/2 cup cherry tomatoes, halved
- 1/4 cup of basil pesto (bought from a store or homemade)
- 2 tablespoons grated Parmesan cheese
- 1 tablespoon olive oil
- Salt and pepper to taste
- Fresh basil leaves for garnish

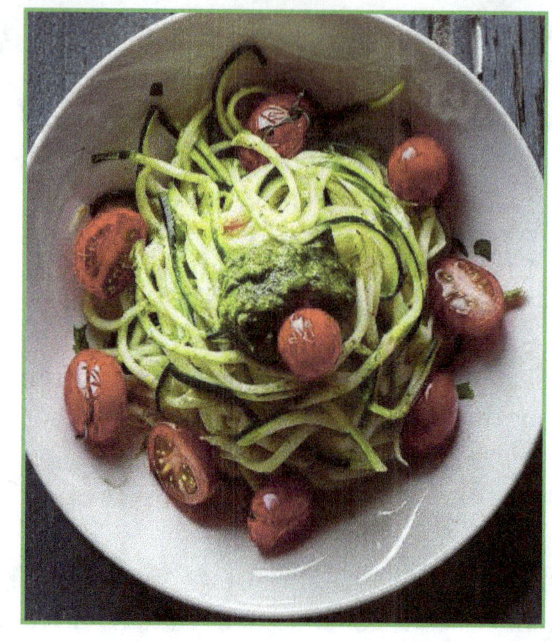

Directions:

1. In a medium-sized pan, heat the olive oil.
2. Add spiralized zucchini noodles to the pan and sauté for 2-3 minutes until just tender.
3. Add cherry tomatoes to the pan and cook for another 1-2 minutes.
4. Stir in basil pesto and toss everything together until noodles and tomatoes are coated.
5. Season with salt and pepper to taste.
6. Take from heat and put it in a serving dish.
7. Sprinkle grated Parmesan cheese on top and garnish with fresh basil leaves.
8. Serve warm.

Nutritional information:

Calories: 250

Protein: 6g

Carbohydrates: 10g

Fiber: 3g

Fat: 20g

Ingredients:

- 2 oak squash, halved, and remove the seeds.
- 1 cup cooked quinoa
- 1/2 cup dried cranberries
- 1/4 cup chopped pecans
- 1/4 cup crumbled goat cheese
- 2 tablespoons maple syrup
- 1 tablespoon olive oil
- 1 teaspoon ground cinnamon
- Salt and pepper to taste

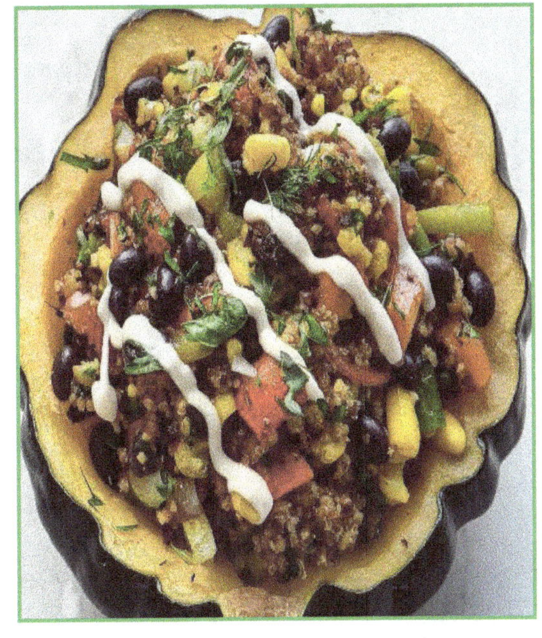

Directions:

1. Preheat oven to 375°F (190°C).
2. Place acorn squash halves on a baking sheet, cut-side up.
3. Drizzle olive oil and maple syrup over each squash half.
4. Sprinkle ground cinnamon, salt, and pepper evenly.
5. Roast in the preheated oven for about 30-35 minutes or until squash is fork-tender.
6. In a bowl, combine cooked quinoa, dried cranberries, chopped pecans, and crumbled goat cheese.
7. Remove squash from the oven and fill each half with the quinoa mixture.
8. Return stuffed squash to the oven and bake for an additional 10 minutes until filling is heated through and cheese is melted.
9. Serve hot as a delicious and nutritious lunch.

Nutritional information:

Calories: 320

Protein: 8g

Carbohydrates: 50g

Fiber: 7g

Fat: 12g

Ingredients:

- 4 large red peppers, halved with seeds removed
- 1 cup quinoa, cooked
- 1 can (15 oz) black beans, drained and rinsed
- 1 cup corn kernels (fresh or frozen)
- 1/2 cup diced tomatoes
- 1/4 cup chopped cilantro
- 1 teaspoon ground cumin
- 1 teaspoon chili powder
- Salt and pepper to taste
- 1/2 cup shredded cheddar cheese (optional)

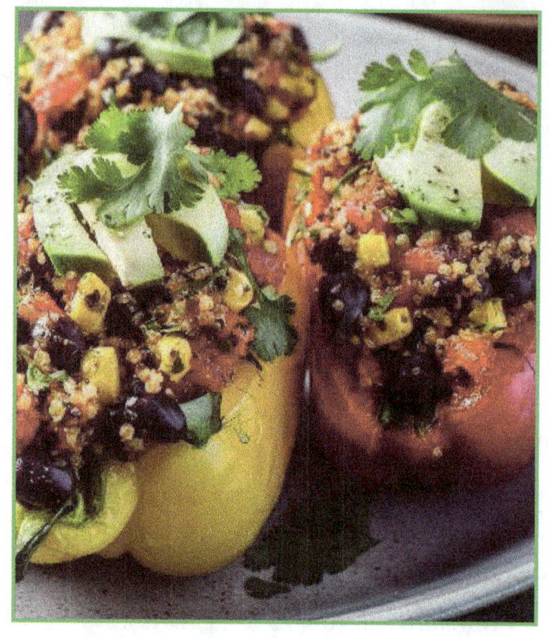

Directions:

1. Preheat oven to 375°F (190°C).
2. In a bowl, combine cooked quinoa, black beans, corn kernels, diced tomatoes, chopped cilantro, ground cumin, chili powder, salt, and pepper.
3. Mix everything until well combined.
4. Fill each bell pepper half with the quinoa mixture.
5. Place stuffed peppers on a baking dish.
6. Optionally, sprinkle shredded cheddar cheese on top of each stuffed pepper.
7. Cover the baking dish with foil and bake in the preheated oven for 25-30 minutes.
8. Remove foil and bake for an additional 5 minutes until cheese is melted and bubbly.
9. Serve hot.

Nutritional information:

Calories: 280

Protein: 12g

Carbohydrates: 45g

Fiber: 10g

Fat: 6g

Ingredients:

- 1 can (5 oz) tuna, drained
- 1/4 cup diced celery
- 1/4 cup diced red onion
- 2 tablespoons plain Greek yogurt
- 1 tablespoon lemon juice
- 1 teaspoon Dijon mustard
- Salt and pepper to taste
- Lettuce leaves for wrapping (such as romaine or butter lettuce)
- Sliced avocado (optional)
- Tomato slices (optional)

Directions:

1. In a bowl, combine drained tuna, diced celery, diced red onion, Greek yogurt, lemon juice, Dijon mustard, salt, and pepper.
2. Mix until well combined.
3. Spoon the tuna salad onto lettuce leaves.
4. Add sliced avocado and tomato slices if desired.
5. Roll up the lettuce leaves to form wraps.
6. Serve immediately.

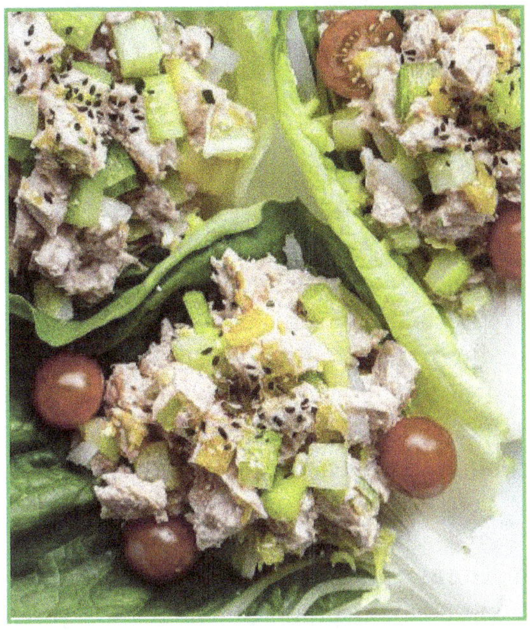

Nutritional information:

Calories: 220

Protein: 25g

Carbohydrates: 5g

Fiber: 2g

Fat: 10g

Ingredients:

- 8 oz beef sirloin, thinly sliced
- 2 cups of mixed veggies (broccoli, peppers, and snap peas).
- 2 tablespoons low-sodium soy sauce
- 1 tablespoon of oyster sauce
- 1 tablespoon of hoisin sauce
- 1 tablespoon cornstarch
- 1 tablespoon sesame oil
- 2 cloves garlic, minced
- 1 teaspoon grated ginger
- 2 green onions, chopped
- Salt and pepper to taste
- Cooked brown rice for serving

Directions:

1. Marinate the thinly sliced beef in a mixture of the following: soy sauce, oyster sauce, hoisin sauce, cornstarch, salt, and pepper. Let it sit for 15-20 minutes.
2. Heat sesame oil in a wok or large skillet over high heat.
3. Add minced garlic and grated ginger, stir-fry for a few seconds until fragrant.
4. Add marinated beef to the wok and stir-fry until browned and cooked through.
5. Add mixed vegetables and continue stir-frying until vegetables are tender-crisp.
6. Sprinkle chopped green onions on top and toss everything together.
7. Adjust seasoning if needed.
8. Serve the beef stir-fry over cooked brown rice.

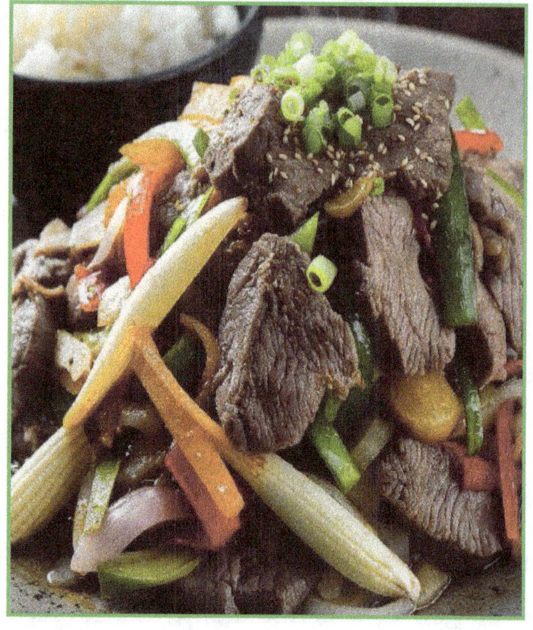

Nutritional information:

Calories: 320

Protein: 25g

Carbohydrates: 30g

Fiber: 6g

Fat: 12g

Ingredients:

- 6 oz salmon fillet
- 1 cup broccoli florets
- 1 cup cauliflower florets
- 1/2 cup sliced carrots
- 1 tablespoon olive oil
- Lemon slices for garnish
- Salt and pepper to taste

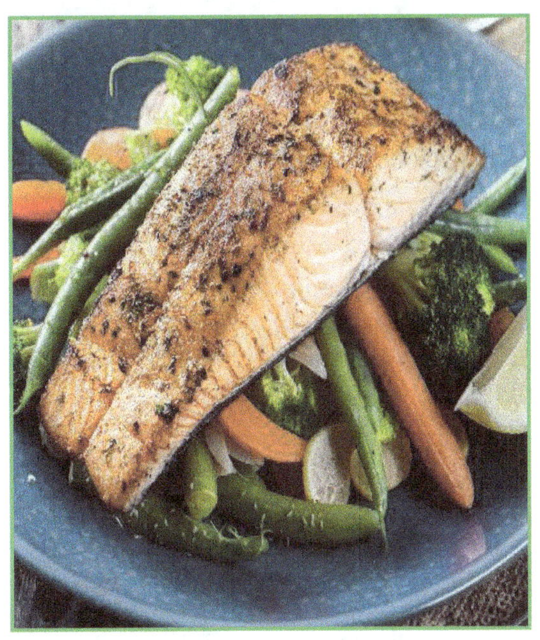

Directions:

1. Preheat the grill pan over a slightly-high heat.
2. Season salmon fillet with salt, pepper, and a drizzle of olive oil.
3. Grill salmon for about 4-5 minutes per side or until cooked through.
4. In the meantime, steam broccoli, cauliflower, and carrots until tender.
5. Arrange steamed vegetables on a plate.
6. Place grilled salmon on top of the vegetables.
7. Dish with lemon slices prior to serving.

Nutritional information:

Calories: 320

Protein: 30g

Carbohydrates: 10g

Fiber: 4g

Fat: 18g

Ingredients:

- 1 cup dried lentils, rinsed
- 4 cups low-sodium vegetable broth
- 1 cup diced carrots
- 1 cup diced celery
- 1 cup diced potatoes
- 1/2 cup diced onion
- 2 cloves garlic, minced
- 1 teaspoon dried thyme
- Salt and pepper to taste
- Fresh parsley for garnish

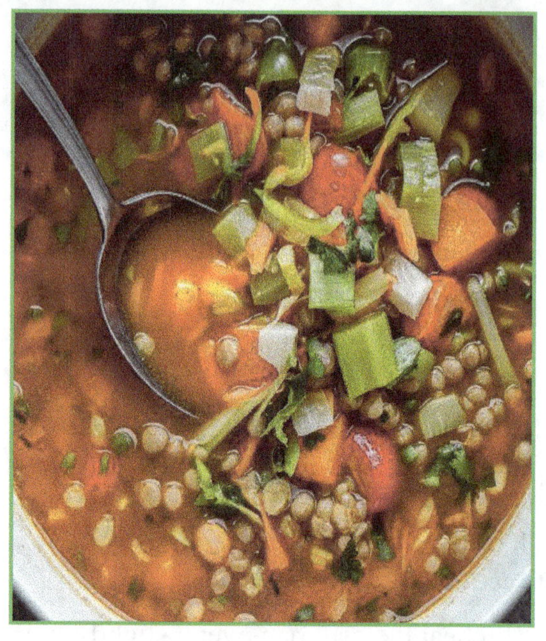

Directions:

1. In a pot, combine lentils, vegetable broth, carrots, celery, potatoes, onion, garlic, and thyme.

2. Bring to a boil, then reduce heat and simmer uncovered for 25-30 minutes or until lentils and vegetables are tender.

3. Season with pepper and salt to enrich the taste.

4. Garnish with fresh parsley before serving.

Nutritional information:

Calories: 280

Protein: 15g

Carbohydrates: 45g

Fiber: 12g

Fat: 2g

Ingredients:

- 4 oz grilled chicken breast, sliced
- 2 cups romaine lettuce, chopped
- 1/4 cup cherry tomatoes, halved
- 1/4 cup sliced cucumber
- 2 tablespoons grated Parmesan cheese
- 2 tablespoons Caesar dressing (low-fat)
- Croutons (optional)
- Salt and pepper to taste

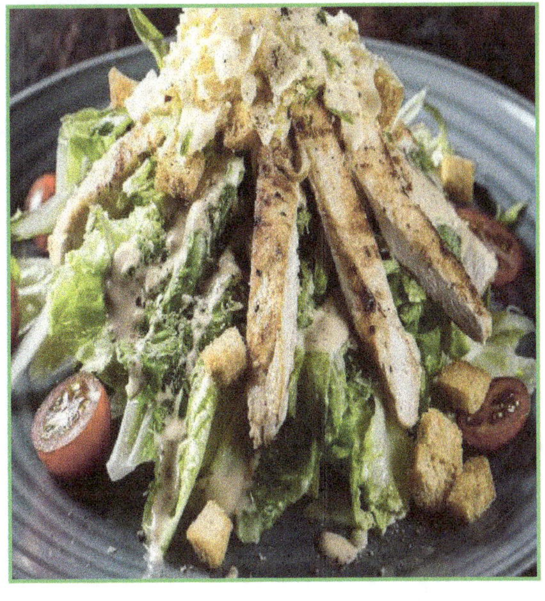

Directions:

1. In a large bowl, combine romaine lettuce, cherry tomatoes, cucumber, and Parmesan cheese.

2. Add grilled chicken slices on top.

3. Drizzle Caesar dressing over the salad.

4. Stir everything together till they uniformly coated.

5. Season with salt and pepper to taste.

6. Optionally, add croutons for added crunch.

7. Serve immediately.

Nutritional information:

Calories: 280

Protein: 30g

Carbohydrates: 10g

Fiber: 4g

Fat: 12g

Ingredients:

- 1 pre-made whole wheat pie crust
- 4 large eggs
- 1 cup chopped spinach
- 1 cup sliced mushrooms
- 1/2 cup shredded Swiss cheese
- 1/2 cup of milk
- 1/4 cup diced onion
- 1 tablespoon olive oil
- Salt and pepper to taste

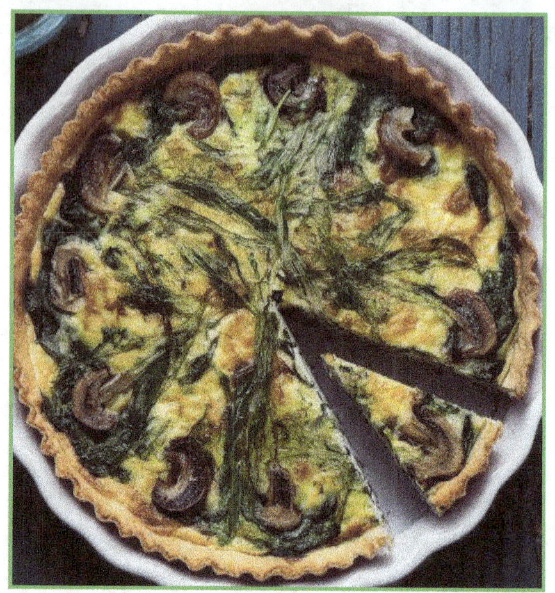

Directions:

1. Preheat oven to 375°F (190°C).
2. In a saucepan, heat the olive oil on medium heat.
3. Add diced onion and sauté until translucent.
4. Add sliced mushrooms and cook until tender.
5. Add minced spinach and boil until softened. Remove it from heat.
6. In a bowl, whisk together eggs, milk, salt, and pepper.
7. Place the pre-made pie crust in a pie dish.
8. Spread the cooked vegetables evenly over the pie crust.
9. Sprinkle shredded Swiss cheese on top of the vegetables.
10. Pour the egg mixture over the vegetables and cheese.
11. Bake in the oven that has been preheated for 30-35 minutes, up to the time the quiche has set and turned golden brown.
12. Let it cool slightly before slicing and serving.

Nutritional information:

Calories: 280

Protein: 12g

Carbohydrates: 20g

Fiber: 2g

Fat: 16g

Ingredients:

- 1 cup of dried green lentils, washed.
- 4 cups low-sodium vegetable broth
- 1 cup diced carrots
- 1 cup diced celery
- 1 cup diced potatoes
- 1/2 cup diced onion
- 2 cloves garlic, minced
- 1 teaspoon of dried thyme
- 1 teaspoon smoked paprika
- Salt and pepper to taste
- Fresh parsley for garnish

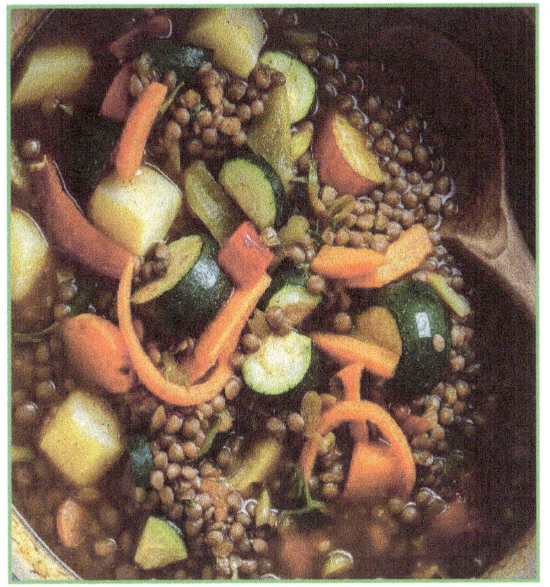

Directions:

1. In a large pot, combine dried lentils, vegetable broth, diced carrots, celery, potatoes, onion, garlic, dried thyme, smoked paprika, salt, and pepper.

2. Bring to a boil, then reduce heat to low and simmer uncovered for about 25-30 minutes or until lentils and vegetables are tender.

3. 3. Stir occasionally and add more broth if needed.

4. Adjust seasoning to taste.

5. Dish while warm and garnished with freshly chopped parsley.

Nutritional information:

Calories: 280

Protein: 15g

Carbohydrates: 50g

Fiber: 12g

Fat: 2g

PHASE 3
HIGH-FIBER MAINTENANCE DIET
(FOR LONG-TERM PREVENTION)

CHAPTER 6

HIGH-FIBER MAINTENANCE DIET (FOR LONG-TERM PREVENTION) RECIPES

CHIA SEED PUDDING

Ingredients:

- 3 tablespoons chia seeds
- 1 cup unsweetened almond milk
- 1 tablespoon of either honey or maple syrup
- 1/2 teaspoon vanilla extract
- Fresh berries for topping
- Salt and pepper to enrich taste

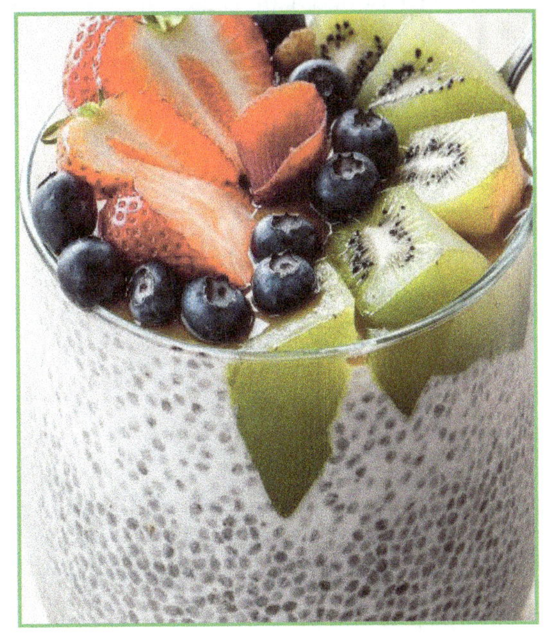

Directions:

1. In a bowl, combine the chia seeds, almond milk, either honey or maple syrup, and vanilla essence.
2. Stir well and let it sit for 10 minutes, then stir again to avoid clumping.
3. Cover the bowl and refrigerate overnight or for at least 4 hours until the mixture thickens into a pudding-like consistency.
4. Serve chilled, topped with fresh berries.

Nutritional information:

Calories: 150

Protein: 4g

Carbohydrates: 15g

Fiber: 10g

Fat: 8g

Ingredients:

- 1 cup of quinoa, cooked and allow to cooled
- 1 can (15 ounces) of rinsed and drained black beans
- 1 cup diced red peppers or (any color)
- 1/2 cup diced cucumber
- 1/4 cup chopped fresh cilantro
- 2 tablespoons olive oil
- 2 tablespoons lime juice
- 1 teaspoon ground cumin
- Salt and pepper to taste

Directions:

1. In a large bowl, combine cooked quinoa, black beans, diced bell peppers, diced cucumber, and chopped cilantro.

2. In a small bowl, whisk together olive oil, lime juice, ground cumin, salt, and pepper.

3. Drizzle the dressing over the quinoa mixture and toss to incorporate well.

4. Serve chilled.

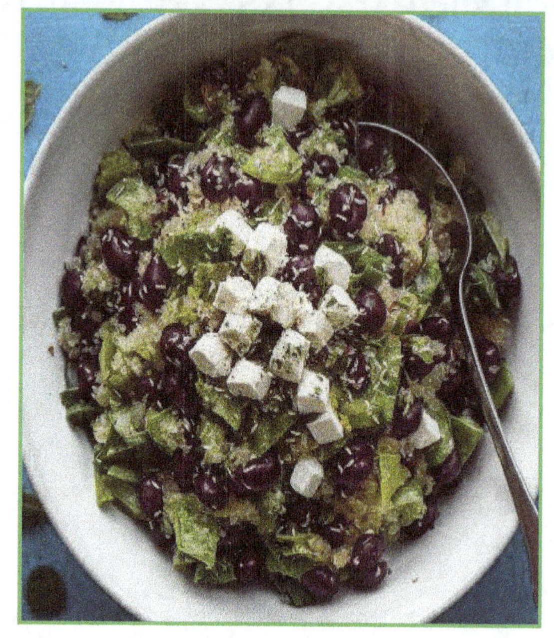

Nutritional information:

Calories: 280

Protein: 10g

Carbohydrates: 35g

Fiber: 8g

Fat: 10g

Ingredients:
- 1 cup of dried green lentils and washed very well.
- 2 cups vegetable broth
- 2 sweet potatoes, peeled clean and cut into cubes.
- 1 can (15 oz) diced tomatoes
- 1 can (15 oz) coconut milk
- 1 onion, chopped
- 2 cloves garlic, minced
- 1 tablespoon curry powder
- 1 teaspoon ground turmeric
- Salt and pepper to taste
- Fresh cilantro for garnish
- Cooked brown rice for serving

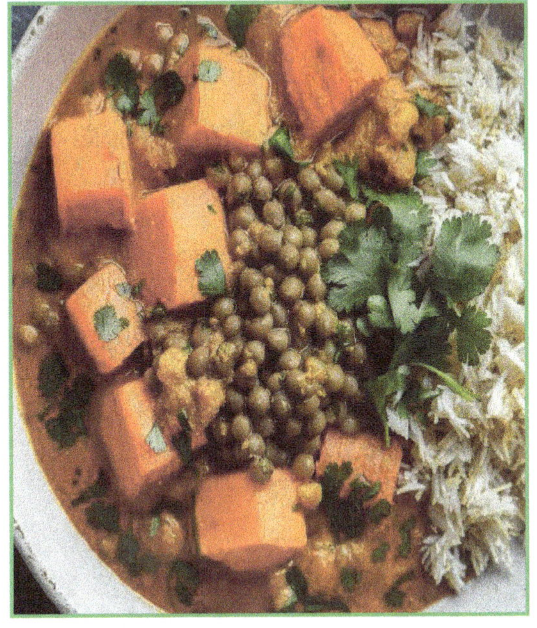

Directions:

1. In a large pot, combine dried lentils, vegetable broth, sweet potatoes, diced tomatoes (with juices), chopped onion, minced garlic, curry powder, ground turmeric, salt, and pepper.

2. Bring to a boil, then reduce heat and simmer for about 20-25 minutes or until lentils and sweet potatoes are tender.

3. Stir in coconut milk and simmer for an additional 5 minutes.

4. Adjust seasoning if needed.

5. Dish the curry onto cooked brown rice and sprinkle with fresh cilantro.

Nutritional information:

Calories: 350

Protein: 12g

Carbohydrates: 45g

Fiber: 12g

Fat: 15g

Ingredients:

- 4 boneless, skinless chicken breasts
- 2 cups chopped spinach
- 1 cup sliced mushrooms
- 1/4 cup diced onion
- 2 cloves garlic, minced
- 1/4 cup shredded mozzarella cheese
- 1 tablespoon olive oil
- Salt and pepper to taste

Directions:

1. Preheat oven to 375°F (190°C).
2. In a saucepan, heat the olive oil with little medium heat.
3. Add diced onion and minced garlic, sauté until softened.
4. Add chopped spinach and sliced mushrooms, cook until vegetables are tender and moisture has evaporated.
5. Season with salt and pepper.
6. Butterfly each chicken breast by slicing horizontally through the middle, but not cutting all the way through.
7. Stuff each chicken breast with the spinach and mushroom mixture.
8. Sprinkle shredded mozzarella cheese over the stuffing.
9. Secure the chicken breasts with toothpicks or tie with kitchen twine.
10. Place stuffed chicken breasts on a baking sheet and bake in the preheated oven for 25-30 minutes or until chicken is cooked through and juices run clear.
11. Remove toothpicks or twine before serving.

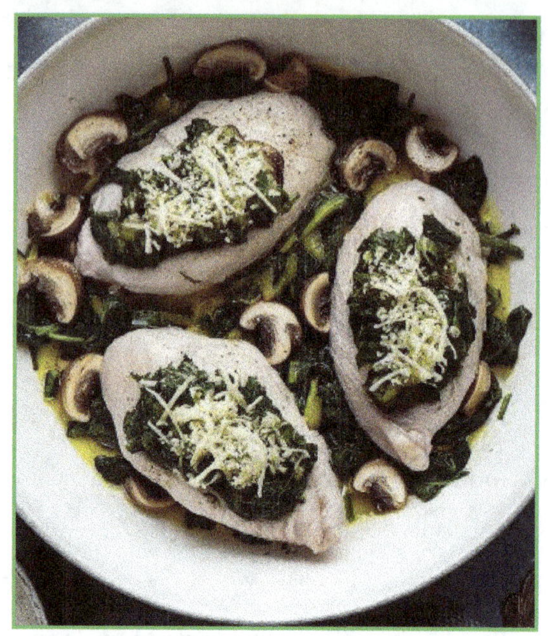

Nutritional information:

Calories: 320

Protein: 30g

Carbohydrates: 10g

Fiber: 3g

Fat: 18g

Ingredients:

- 1 cup Greek yogurt (unsweetened)
- 1/2 cup of a variety of berries (strawberries, blueberries and raspberries)
- 1/4 cup granola (choose a high-fiber variety)
- 1 tablespoon of honey (optional).

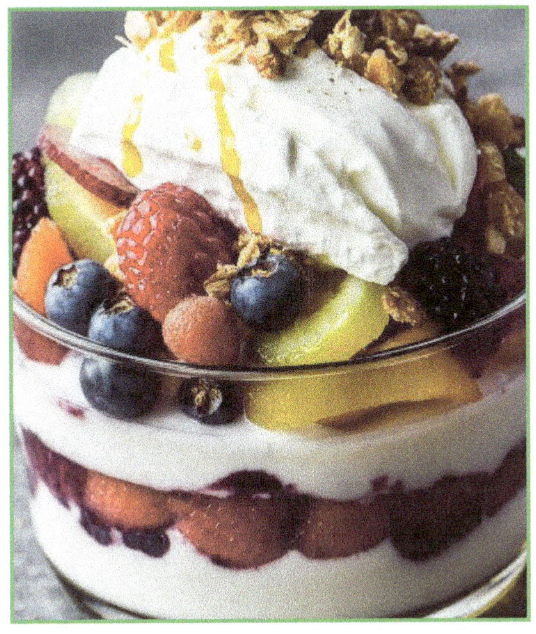

Directions:

1. In a glass or dish, combine the Greek yogurt, mixed berries, and granola.
2. Drizzle honey or maple syrup on top if desired.
3. Repeat the layers if making multiple servings.
4. Serve chilled as a healthy and filling snack or breakfast.

Nutritional information:

Calories: 250

Protein: 15g

Carbohydrates: 35g

Fiber: 6g

Fat: 8g

Ingredients:

- 1 large whole grain wrap or tortilla
- 2 tablespoons hummus
- 1/4 cup shredded carrots
- 1/4 cup thinly sliced cucumber
- 1/4 cup baby spinach leaves
- 1/4 cup of diced peppers of any color
- 1/4 cup avocado slices
- Salt and pepper to taste

Directions:

1. Spread hummus evenly on the whole grain wrap.
2. Layer shredded carrots, sliced cucumber, baby spinach leaves, diced bell peppers, and avocado slices on the wrap.
3. Season with salt and pepper.
4. Roll up the wrap tightly, cut in half if desired, and serve.

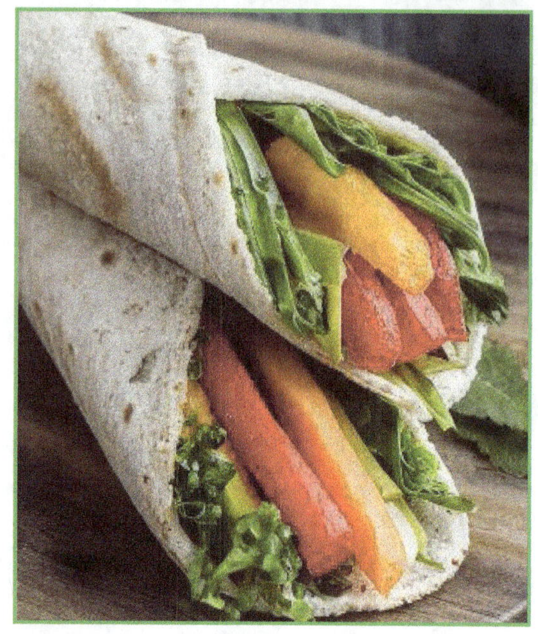

Nutritional information:

Calories: 300

Protein: 8g

Carbohydrates: 35g

Fiber: 9g

Fat:

Ingredients:

- 1 cup of quinoa, cooked
- 1 medium sweet potato, cubed
- 1 cup of broccoli florets
- 1 cup cauliflower florets
- 1 cup of diced peppers of any color
- 1/4 cup chopped red onion
- 2 tablespoons olive oil
- 1 teaspoon smoked paprika
- 1/2 teaspoon garlic powder
- Salt and pepper to taste
- Fresh parsley for garnish

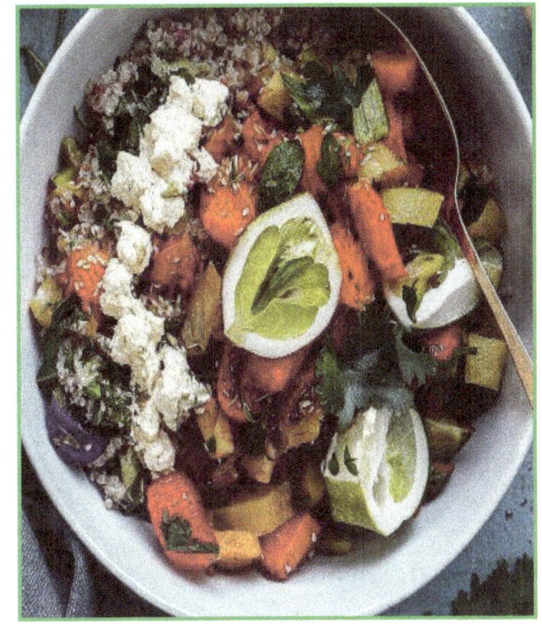

Directions:

1. Preheat oven to 400°F (200°C)
2. In a large bowl, toss sweet potato cubes, broccoli florets, cauliflower florets, diced bell peppers, and red onion with olive oil, smoked paprika, garlic powder, salt, and pepper until evenly coated.
3. Lay the greens out in a single layer on a baking sheet.
4. Roast in the preheated oven for 20-25 minutes or until vegetables are tender and lightly browned.
5. Divide the cooked quinoa into bowls and top with the roasted vegetables.
6. Sprinkle with freshly chopped parsley and serve.

Nutritional information:

Calories: 320

Protein: 8g

Carbohydrates: 50g

Fiber: 10g

Fat: 10g

Ingredients:
- 1 cup of dried green or brown lentils, rinsed and drained
- 4 cups vegetable broth
- 1 onion, chopped
- 2 carrots, diced
- 2 celery stalks, diced
- 1 can (15 oz) diced tomatoes
- 2 cloves garlic, minced
- 1 teaspoon of ground cumin
- 1 teaspoon dried thyme
- Salt and pepper to taste
- Fresh parsley for garnish

Directions:

1. In a large pot, mix the dried lentils, vegetable broth, chopped onion, diced carrots, diced celery, diced tomatoes (with juices), minced garlic, ground cumin, dried thyme, salt, and pepper.

2. Boil and then reduce heat and simmer covered for about 25-30 minutes or until lentils and vegetables are tender.

3. Adjust seasoning if needed.

4. Serve warm and sprinkle with fresh parsley.

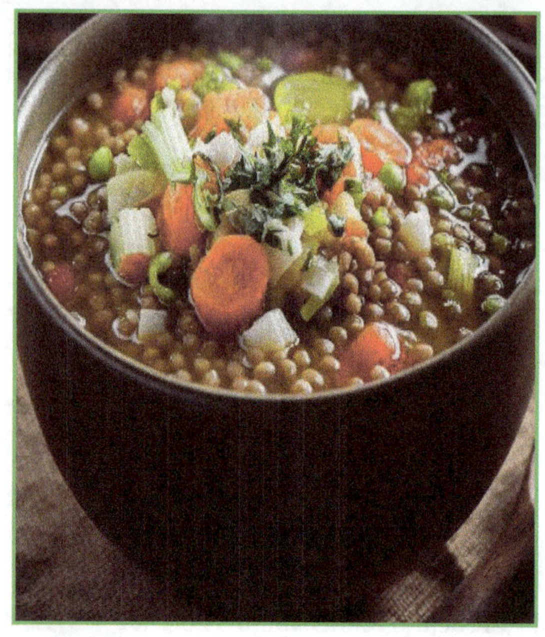

Nutritional information:

Calories: 280

Protein: 15g

Carbohydrates: 45g

Fiber: 12g

Fat: 2g

Ingredients:

- 1 can (15 ounce) of chickpeas, rinsed well and drained
- 1 cup diced cucumber
- 1 cup halved cherry tomatoes
- 1/4 cup diced red onion
- 1/4 cup chopped fresh parsley
- 2 tablespoons extra virgin olive oil
- 1 tablespoon lemon juice
- 1 teaspoon dried oregano
- Salt and pepper to enrich taste
- Crumbled feta cheese (optional)

Directions:

1. In a large bowl, mix the chickpeas, diced cucumber, halved cherry tomatoes, diced red onion, and chopped parsley.

2. In a small bowl, whisk together olive oil, lemon juice, dried oregano, salt, and pepper.

3. Splash the dressing across the blended chickpeas and toss to coat evenly.

4. If using, sprinkle crumbled feta cheese on top.

5. Serve chilled as a refreshing salad.

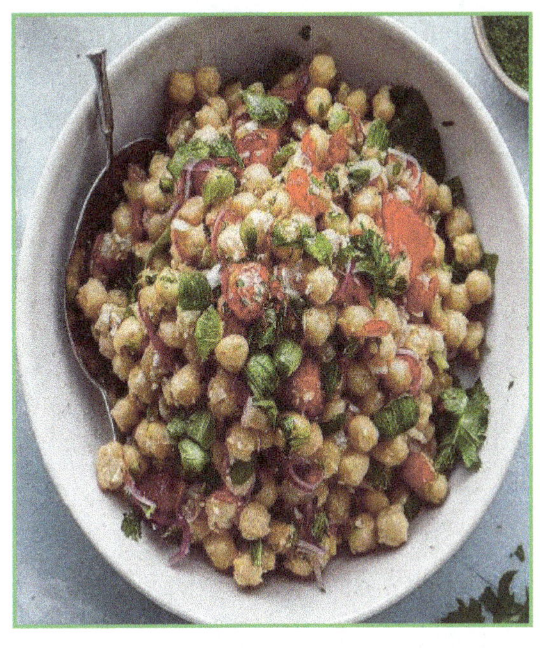

Nutritional information:

Calories: 280

Protein: 10g

Carbohydrates: 35g

Fiber: 10g

Fat: 14g

Ingredients:

- 1 large whole grain tortilla
- 1/2 cup of grilled veggies (bell peppers, zucchini, eggplant)
- 1/4 cup hummus
- Handful of baby spinach leaves
- Salt and pepper to enrich the taste

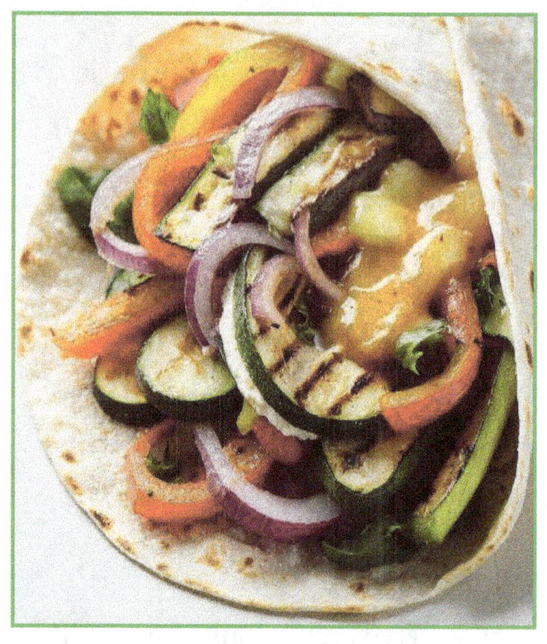

Directions:

1. Spread hummus evenly on the whole grain wrap.
2. Layer grilled vegetables and baby spinach leaves on top of the hummus.
3. Season with pepper and salt to taster.
4. Roll up the wrap tightly, slice if desired, and serve.

Nutritional information:

Calories: 250

Protein: 8g

Carbohydrates: 35g

Fiber: 9g

Fat: 10g

Ingredients:

- 1 cup of cooked lentils
- 1 tablespoon of olive oil
- 1 small onion, diced
- 2 cloves garlic, minced
- 1 teaspoon ground cumin
- 1 teaspoon chili powder
- 1/2 teaspoon paprika
- Pepper and Salt to enrich the taste
- 8 small corn tortillas
- Toppings: diced tomatoes, shredded lettuce, avocado slices, salsa, Greek yogurt (optional)

Directions:

1. Heat olive oil in a saucepan over little medium heat.
2. Sauté sliced onion and minced garlic until tender.
3. Stir in cooked lentils, ground cumin, chili powder, paprika, salt, and pepper.
4. Cook for a few minutes until heated through and flavors are blended.
5. Warm corn tortillas in a separate skillet or microwave.
6. Spoon the lentil mixture onto each tortilla.
7. Add desired toppings such as diced tomatoes, shredded lettuce, avocado slices, salsa, and Greek yogurt.
8. Serve the lentil tacos warm.

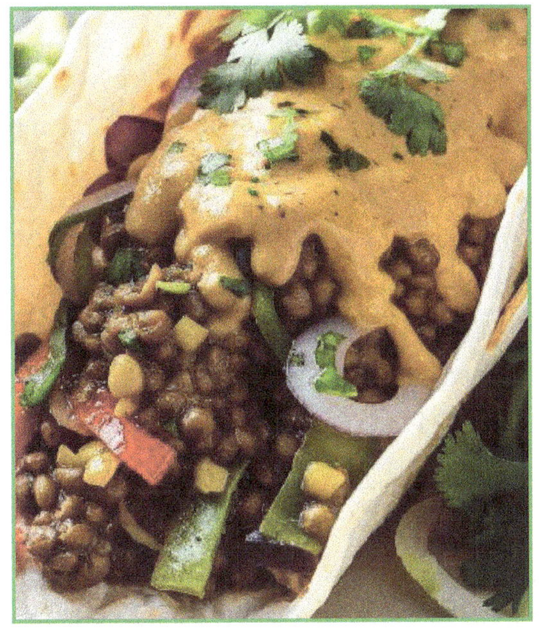

Nutritional information:

Calories: 300

Protein: 12g

Carbohydrates: 45g

Fiber: 10g

Fat: 8g

Ingredients:

- 1 cup of quinoa, cooked it and leave to chilled
- 1 can (15 ounce) of black beans, cleaned and sapped
- 1 ripe mango, sliced
- 1/2 cup diced red bell pepper
- 1/4 cup chopped fresh cilantro
- 2 tablespoons lime juice
- 2 tablespoons extra virgin olive oil
- Salt and pepper to taste

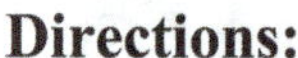

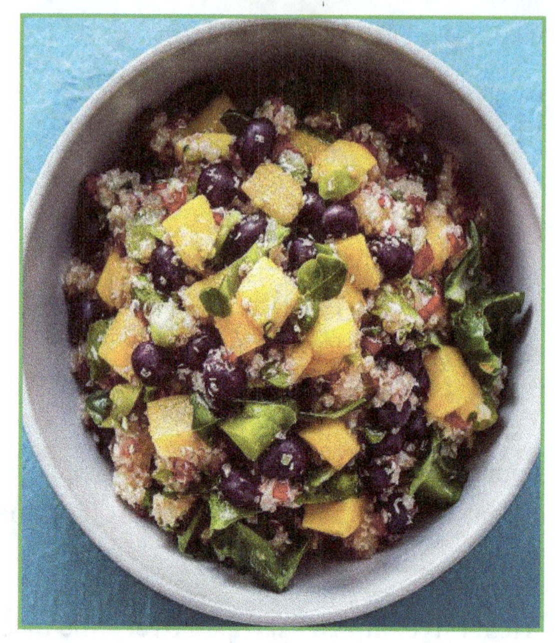

Directions:

1. In a large mixing dish, combine cooked quinoa, black beans, diced mango, diced red bell pepper, and freshly chopped cilantro evenly.

2. In a small bowl, whisk the mixture of lime juice, olive oil, salt, and pepper together.

3. Pour the dressing over the quinoa mixture and toss to mix evenly.

4. Adjust seasoning if needed.

5. Serve the mango and black bean quinoa salad chilled as a refreshing side dish or light meal.

Nutritional information:

Calories: 280

Protein: 10g

Carbohydrates: 45g

Fiber: 8g

Fat: 8g

Ingredients:

- 1 can (15 ounce) chickpeas, cleaned and sapped
- 1/4 cup of fresh chopped parsley
- 1/4 cup of chopped red onion
- 2 cloves garlic, minced
- 2 heaping tablespoons of pure wheat flour
- 1 teaspoon ground cumin
- 1 teaspoon ground coriander
- 1/2 teaspoon baking powder
- Salt and pepper to taste
- 2 tablespoons olive oil

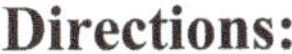

Directions:

1. Preheat oven to 375°F (190°C). Line a baking sheet with parchment paper.
2. In a food processor, mix chickpeas, chopped parsley, chopped red onion, minced garlic, whole wheat flour, ground cumin, ground coriander, baking powder, salt, and pepper.
3. Pulse until the mixture comes together but still has some texture.
4. Shape the mixture into small patties and place them on the prepared baking sheet.
5. Brush the patties lightly with olive oil.
6. Bake in a preheated oven for 20-25 minutes, tossing halfway through, till the inside of the falafel is golden and crispy.
7. Serve the baked falafel patties with whole wheat pita bread, hummus, and fresh vegetables.

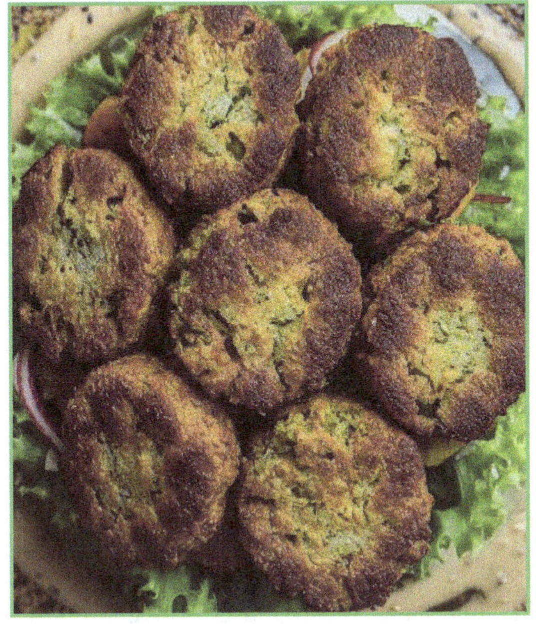

Nutritional information:

Calories: 250

Protein: 10g

Carbohydrates: 35g

Fiber: 8g

Fat: 10g

Ingredients:

- 2 cups of broccoli florets
- 1 can (15 ounce) of chickpeas, cleaned and sapped
- 1 slice of bell pepper
- 1/2 cup sliced carrots
- 2 cloves of garlic and mince it
- 2 tablespoons low-sodium soy sauce
- 1 tablespoon hoisin sauce
- 1 tablespoon sesame oil
- 1 teaspoon grated ginger
- Red pepper flakes (optional)
- Cooked brown rice for serving

Directions:

1. Heat sesame oil in a large saucepan with medium heat.
2. Sauté minced garlic and grated ginger for 1 minute, until they become aromatic.
3. Add broccoli florets, sliced bell pepper, sliced carrots, and chickpeas to the skillet.
4. Stir-fry for about 5-7 minutes until vegetables are tender-crisp.
5. In a small bowl, mix together low-sodium soy sauce, hoisin sauce, and red pepper flakes if using.
6. Pour the sauce over the stir-fried vegetables and chickpeas.
7. Toss everything together until well coated and heated through.
8. Serve the broccoli and chickpea stir-fry over cooked brown rice.

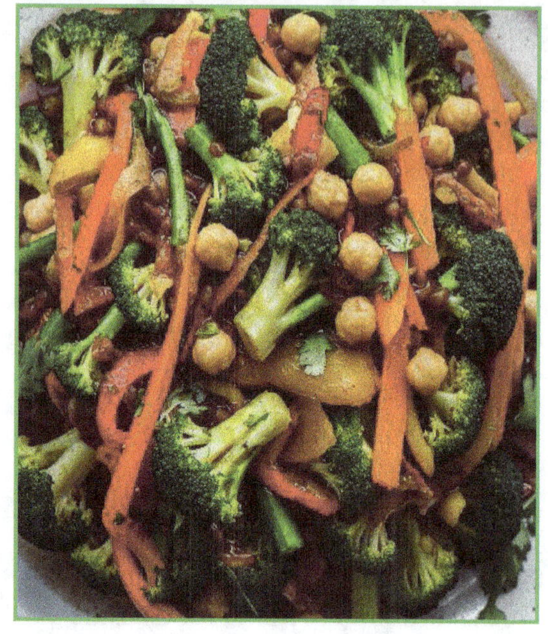

Nutritional information:

Calories: 300

Protein: 12g

Carbohydrates: 45g

Fiber: 10g

Fat: 8g

Ingredients:
- 1 eggplant, cubed
- 2 zucchinis, cubed
- 1 onion, diced
- 1 bell pepper, diced
- 2 cloves garlic, minced
- 1 can (15 oz) diced tomatoes
- 2 tablespoons tomato paste
- 1 teaspoon dried thyme
- 1 teaspoon dried oregano
- Salt and pepper to taste
- Fresh basil for garnish

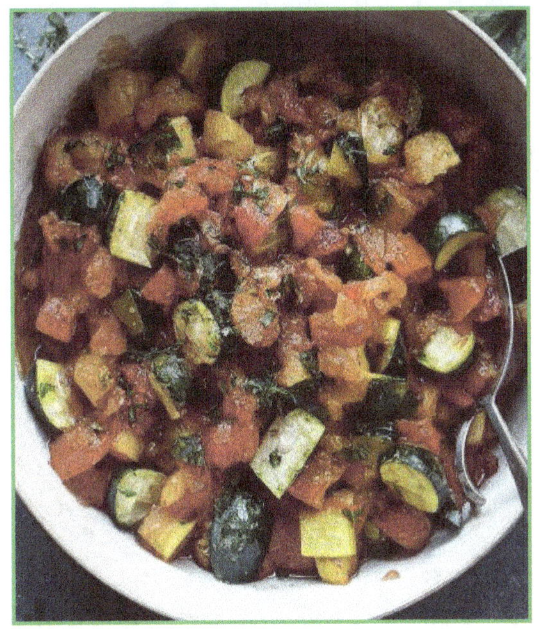

Directions:
1. Heat olive oil in a big pot with medium heat.
2. Sauté sliced onion and minced garlic until tender.
3. Add cubed eggplant and zucchinis to the pot, cook for a few minutes until slightly softened.
4. Stir in diced bell pepper, diced tomatoes (with juices), tomato paste, dried thyme, dried oregano, salt, and pepper.
5. Reduce heat to low, cover, and simmer for about 20-25 minutes, stirring occasionally, until vegetables are tender and flavors are well combined.
6. Adjust seasoning if needed.
7. Serve the eggplant and zucchini ratatouille hot, garnished with fresh basil.

Nutritional information:

Calories: 220

Protein: 6g

Carbohydrates: 35g

Fiber: 12g

Fat: 8g

Ingredients:

- 1 can (15 ounce) of chickpeas, cleaned and drained
- 1/2 cup of fresh chopped parsley
- 1/4 cup of chopped red onion
- 2 cloves of garlic, sliced
- 1 teaspoon ground cumin
- 1 teaspoon ground coriander
- 1/4 teaspoon cayenne pepper (optional)
- Pepper and salt to enrich the taste
- 2 tablespoons olive oil
- Tahini sauce for serving

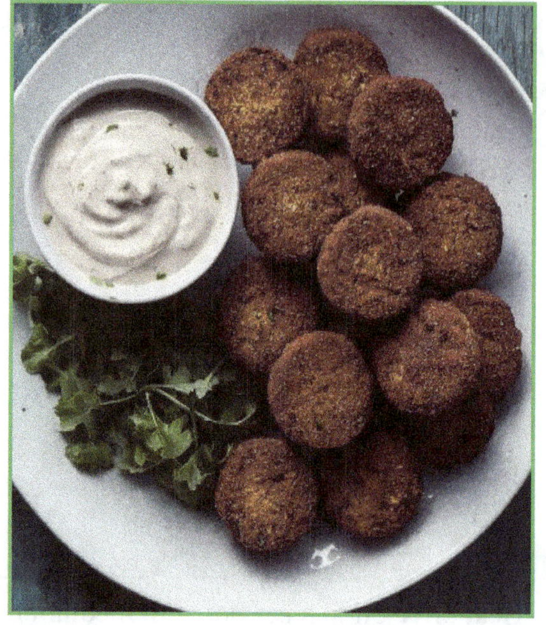

Directions:

1. Preheat the oven to 375°F (190°C). Lay the baking sheet with baking parchment.
2. In a food processor, combine chickpeas, chopped parsley, red onion, minced garlic, ground cumin, ground coriander, cayenne pepper (if using), salt, and pepper.
3. Pulse until mixture is coarsely ground and holds together when pressed.
4. Shape the mixture into small falafel patties and place them on the prepared baking sheet.
5. Brush the tops of the falafel patties with olive oil.
6. Bake for 20-25 minutes, flipping halfway through, until falafel is golden brown and crispy.
7. Serve the baked falafel with tahini sauce for dipping.

Nutritional information:

Calories: 220

Protein: 8g

Carbohydrates: 30g

Fiber: 8g

Fat: 9g

Ingredients:

- 4 big bell peppers, half it and removed the seeds
- 1 cup cooked lentils
- 1 cup diced mushrooms
- 1/2 cup diced onion
- 2 cloves garlic, minced
- 1 teaspoon dried thyme
- 1 teaspoon smoked paprika
- Salt and pepper to taste
- 1/2 cup shredded mozzarella cheese (optional)

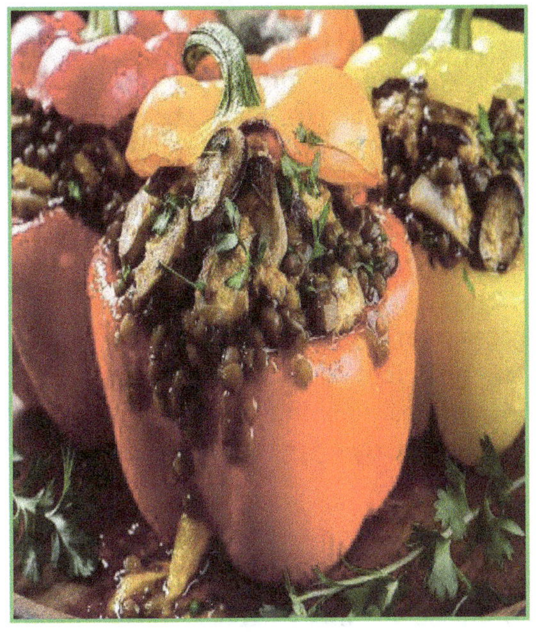

Directions:

1. Preheat oven to 375°F (190°C).
2. In a skillet, sauté diced mushrooms, onion, and minced garlic until softened.
3. Stir in cooked lentils, dried thyme, smoked paprika, salt, and pepper. Boil for a couple of minutes to mix the flavors.
4. Fill each bell pepper half with the lentil and mushroom mixture.
5. Put the filled peppers in a baking pan. If using, sprinkle shredded mozzarella cheese on top of each pepper.
6. Cover the baking dish with foil and bake for 25-30 minutes.
7. Remove the foil and oven for 5 more minutes, till the cheese is melted and bubbling.
8. Serve the stuffed bell peppers hot.

Nutritional information:

Calories: 180

Protein: 8g

Carbohydrates: 30g

Fiber: 8g

Fat: 3g

Ingredients:

- 4 big whole grain tortillas
- 1 can (15 ounce) black beans, cleaned and drained
- 1 cup corn kernels (fresh or frozen)
- 1/2 cup diced red onion
- 1/2 cup diced bell peppers (any color)
- 1 teaspoon ground cumin
- 1 teaspoon chili powder
- 1/2 cup shredded cheddar cheese
- Olive oil for cooking
- Salsa and Greek yogurt for serving

Directions:

1. In a bowl, mix together black beans, corn kernels, diced red onion, diced bell peppers, ground cumin, and chili powder.
2. Heat a non-stick skillet over medium heat and lightly brush with olive oil.
3. Place a tortilla in the skillet and spread a quarter of the bean mixture evenly over half of the tortilla.
4. Sprinkle shredded cheddar cheese on top of the bean mixture.
5. Fold the tortilla in half to cover the filling, creating a quesadilla.
6. Cook for 2-3 minutes per side or until golden brown and cheese is melted.
7. Repeat with remaining tortillas and filling.
8. Cut each quesadilla into wedges and serve with salsa and Greek yogurt.

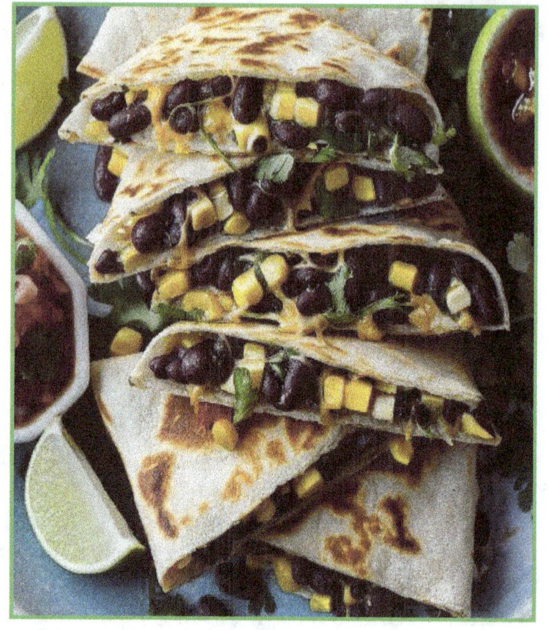

Nutritional information:

Calories: 320

Protein: 12g

Carbohydrates: 45g

Fiber: 10g

Fat: 10g

Ingredients:

- 2 cups cooked brown rice
- 2 cups chopped broccoli florets
- 1 cup of sliced bell peppers of any color
- 1/2 cup of sliced onion
- 2 cloves garlic, minced
- 1/2 cup vegetable broth
- 1/2 cup shredded cheddar cheese
- 2 tablespoons olive oil
- Salt and pepper to taste

Directions:

1. Preheat the oven to 375°F (190°C). Grease the baking pan.
2. In a saucepan, heat olive oil with medium heat.
3. Add diced onion and minced garlic, sauté until translucent.
4. Add chopped broccoli florets and sliced bell peppers, cook until vegetables are tender.
5. In a large bowl, combine cooked brown rice, sautéed vegetables, vegetable broth, shredded cheddar cheese, salt, and pepper. Mix well.
6. Transfer the rice and vegetable mixture to the prepared baking dish.
7. Wrap with foil and place in the oven for 20 minutes.
8. Remove foil and bake for an additional 10 minutes or until the top is golden and bubbly.
9. Let it cool slightly before serving.

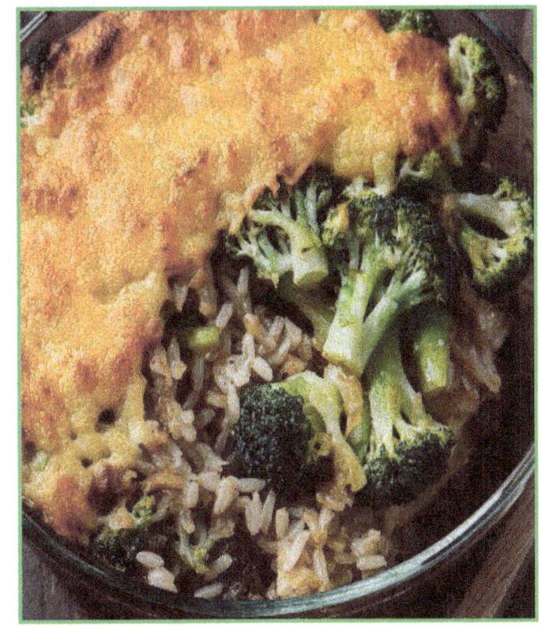

Nutritional information:

Calories: 280

Protein: 10g

Carbohydrates: 40g

Fiber: 8g

Fat: 10g

Ingredients:

- 4 big portion portobello mushrooms with it stems removed.
- 1 cup cooked quinoa
- 1/2 cup diced tomatoes
- 1/2 cup chopped spinach
- 1/4 cup diced red onion
- 1/4 cup crumbled feta cheese
- 2 tablespoons olive oil
- 1 tablespoon balsamic vinegar
- Salt and pepper to taste

Directions:

1. Preheat the oven to 375°F (190°C), then line the surface of the oven with parchment paper.
2. In a bowl, mix cooked quinoa, diced tomatoes, chopped spinach, diced red onion, crumbled feta cheese, olive oil, balsamic vinegar, salt, and pepper.
3. Place portobello mushrooms on the prepared baking sheet.
4. Stuff each mushroom cap with the quinoa mixture.
5. Drizzle a little olive oil on top of each stuffed mushroom.
6. Bake for 20-25 minutes or until mushrooms are tender and filling is heated through.
7. Serve hot as a flavorful and nutritious main dish.

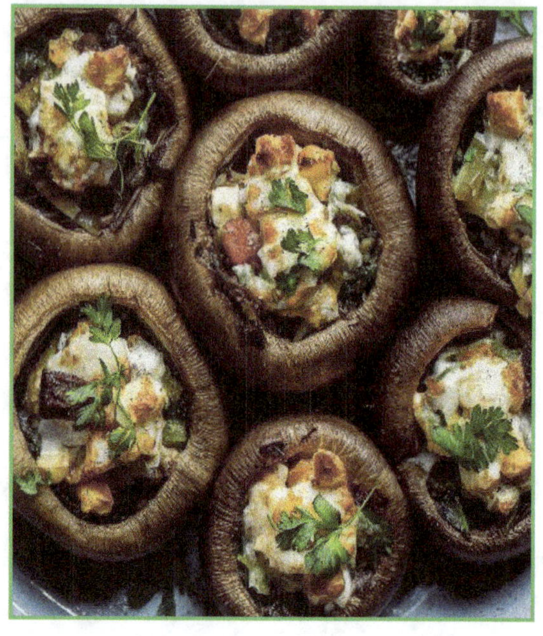

Nutritional information:

Calories: 220

Protein: 9g

Carbohydrates: 25g

Fiber: 6g

Fat: 10g

Ingredients:

- 8 ounce of whole wheat pasta
- 1 cup broccoli florets
- 1 cup sliced bell peppers (any color)
- 1 cup sliced zucchini
- 1/2 cup cherry tomatoes, halved
- 1/4 cup diced red onion
- 2 cloves garlic, minced
- 2 tablespoons olive oil
- 1/4 cup grated Parmesan cheese
- Salt and pepper to taste
- Fresh basil leaves for garnish

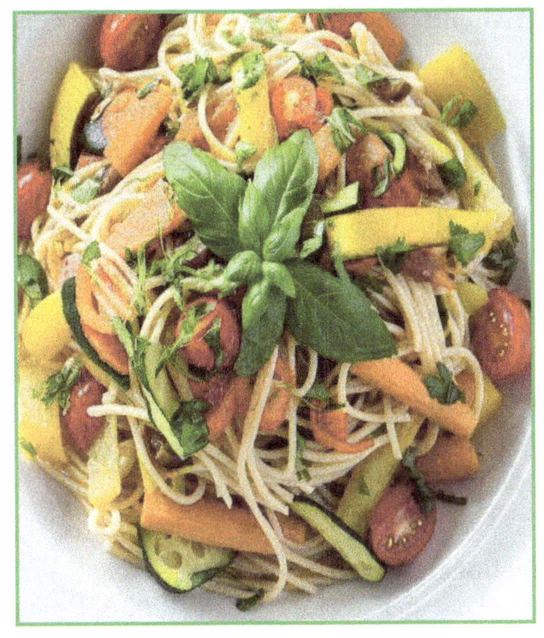

Directions:

1. Cook whole wheat pasta according to package instructions until al dente. Drain and set aside.
2. In a large saucepan, heat olive oil with medium heat.
3. Add sliced garlic and diced red onion, sauté until fragrant.
4. Add broccoli florets, sliced bell peppers, sliced zucchini, and cherry tomatoes to the skillet. Cook until vegetables are tender yet still crisp.
5. Season with pepper and salt to enrich taste.
6. Add cooked pasta to the skillet and toss everything together until well combined.
7. Sprinkle grated Parmesan cheese over the pasta and vegetables.
8. Garnish with fresh basil leaves before serving.
9. Serve hot as a satisfying pasta dish.

Nutritional information:

Calories: 350

Protein: 12g

Carbohydrates: 50g

Fiber: 8g

Fat: 12g

Ingredients:

- 1 big portion of eggplant, sliced into rounds
- 1 cup of whole wheat breadcrumbs
- 1/4 cup grated Parmesan cheese
- 1 teaspoon dried Italian seasoning
- 2 eggs, beaten
- 2 cups of marinara condiment (low sodium)
- 1 cup shredded mozzarella cheese
- Fresh basil leaves for garnish
- Olive oil cooking spray
- Salt and pepper to taste

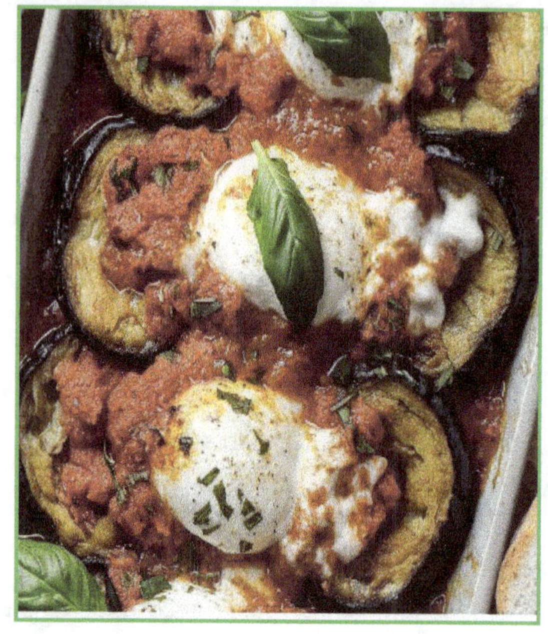

Directions:

1. Preheat the oven to 400°F (200°C) and line a baking sheet with parchment paper.
2. In a shallow bowl, mix whole wheat breadcrumbs, grated Parmesan cheese, dried Italian seasoning, salt, and pepper.
3. Dip eggplant slices into beaten eggs, then coat with the breadcrumb mixture, pressing gently to adhere.
4. Place coated eggplant slices on the prepared baking sheet.
5. Spray the tops of the eggplant slices with olive oil cooking spray.
6. Bake in the preheated oven for 20-25 minutes or until eggplant is tender and coating is crispy.
7. In a baking dish, put a thin layer of marinara condiment.
8. Arrange baked eggplant slices in the dish, overlapping if needed.
9. Top with remaining marinara sauce and shredded mozzarella cheese.
10. Bake for an additional 15 minutes or until cheese is melted and bubbly.
11. Sprinkle with fresh basil leaves before serving.
10. Serve hot as a delicious eggplant Parmesan dish.

Nutritional information:

Calories: 300

Protein: 15g

Carbohydrates: 30g

Fiber: 10g

Fat: 12g

Ingredients:

- 8 ounces of firm tofu, cubed
- 2 cups of mixed veggies (broccoli, bell peppers and snap peas)
- 2 tablespoons low-sodium soy sauce
- 1 tablespoon hoisin sauce
- 1 tablespoon cornstarch
- 1 tablespoon sesame oil
- 2 cloves garlic, minced
- 1 teaspoon grated ginger
- 2 green onions, chopped
- Cooked brown rice for serving
- Salt and pepper to taste

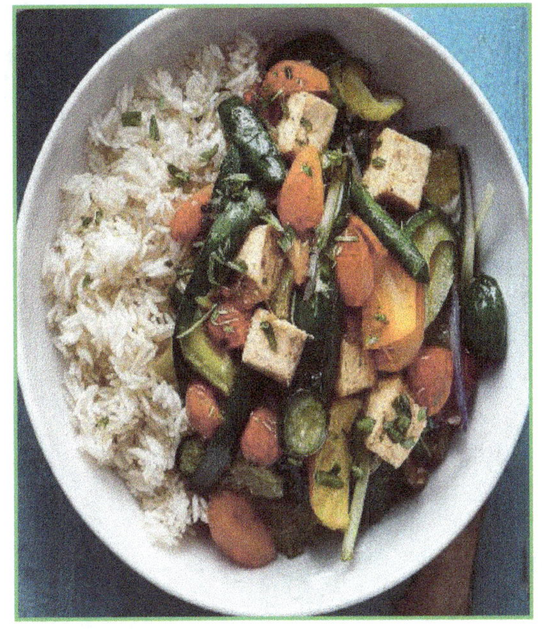

Directions:

1. Press tofu to remove excess water, then cut into cubes.
2. In a bowl, mix together soy sauce, hoisin sauce, cornstarch, grated ginger, salt, and pepper.
3. Heat sesame oil in a wok or large skillet over medium-high heat.
4. Add minced garlic and chopped green onions, sauté for a few seconds.
5. Add cubed tofu to the wok and cook until lightly browned.
6. Add mixed vegetables and stir-fry until vegetables are tender-crisp.
7. Pour the sauce mixture over the tofu and vegetables.
8. Toss everything together until well coated and sauce thickens.
9. Adjust seasoning if needed.
10. Serve the tofu and vegetable stir-fry over cooked brown rice.

Nutritional information:

Calories: 320

Protein: 20g

Carbohydrates: 35g

Fiber: 8g

Fat: 12g

Ingredients:
- 1 big eggplant, sliced
- 1 can (15 ounce) of chickpeas, cleaned and drained
- 1 onion chopped
- 2 cloves of garlic, minced
- 1 tablespoon curry powder
- 1 teaspoon ground turmeric
- 1 teaspoon ground cumin
- 1 can (14 oz) coconut milk
- 1 cup vegetable broth
- 2 tablespoons olive oil
- Salt and pepper to taste
- Fresh cilantro for garnish

Directions:
1. In a big saucepan, heat olive oil with medium heat.
2. Add chopped onion and minced garlic, sauté until softened.
3. Stir in diced eggplant and cook for a few minutes.
4. Add curry powder, ground turmeric, ground cumin, salt, and pepper. Stir to coat the vegetables.
5. Put in the coconut milk and veggie broth. Bring to a simmer.
6. Add drained chickpeas to the pot and stir well.
7. Simmer uncovered for about 20-25 minutes or until eggplant is tender and the curry has thickened.
8. Adjust seasoning if needed.
9. Serve the eggplant and chickpea curry hot, garnished with fresh cilantro.

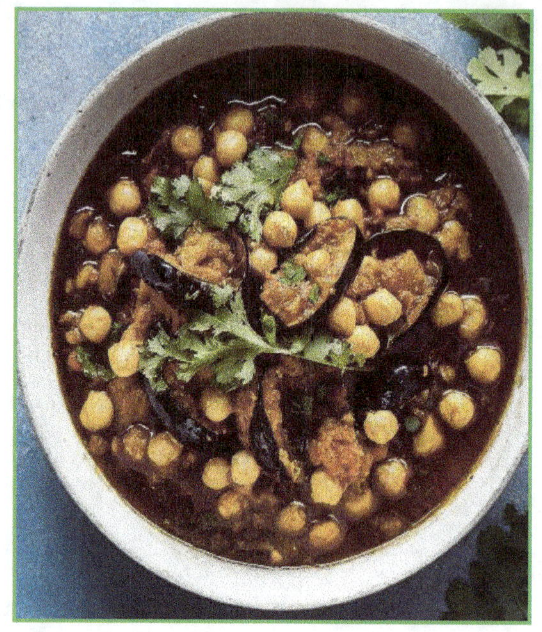

Nutritional information:

Calories: 320

Protein: 10g

Carbohydrates: 35g

Fiber: 12g

Fat: 18g

Ingredients:
- 8 ounce of whole grain pasta (such as penne or fusilli)
- 1 cup of broccoli florets
- 1 cup sliced carrots
- 1 cup cherry tomatoes, halved
- 1/2 cup diced bell peppers (any color)
- 1/4 cup chopped fresh basil
- 2 tablespoons olive oil
- 2 cloves garlic, minced
- Salt and pepper to taste
- Grated Parmesan cheese for serving (optional)

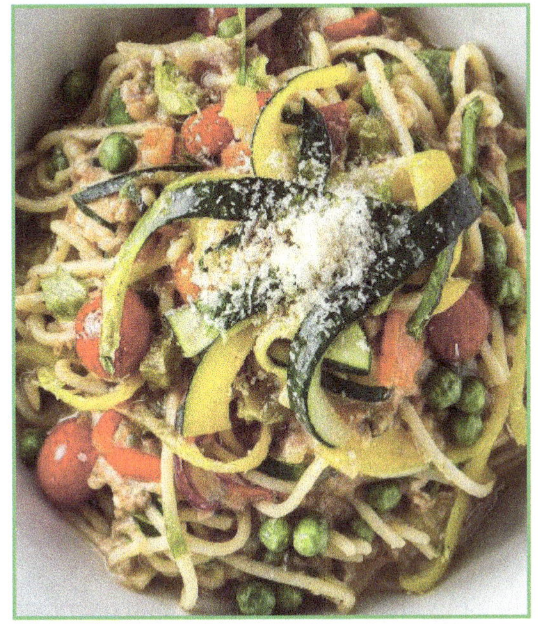

Directions:
1. Cook whole grain pasta according to package instructions until al dente. Drain and set aside.
2. In a large saucepan, heat olive oil with medium heat.
3. Add the minced garlic and cook until fragrant.
4. Add broccoli florets, sliced carrots, cherry tomatoes, and diced bell peppers to the skillet. Cook until vegetables are tender-crisp.
5. Season with pepper and salt to enrich the taste.
6. Add cooked pasta to the skillet and toss to combine with the vegetables.
7. Stir in chopped fresh basil.
8. Remove from heat and serve the pasta primavera hot.
9. If desired, sprinkle grated Parmesan cheese on top before serving.

Nutritional information:

Calories: 350

Protein: 10g

Carbohydrates: 50g

Fiber: 8g

Fat: 12g

Ingredients:

- 1 can (15 ounces) of cleaned and rinsed black beans
- 1 cup of cooked quinoa
- 1/2 cup of sliced bell peppers of any color
- 1/2 cup grated zucchini
- 1/4 cup diced red onion
- 2 cloves garlic, minced
- 1 teaspoon ground cumin
- 1 teaspoon smoked paprika
- 1/4 cup whole wheat breadcrumbs
- 1 egg (or flaxseed meal as a vegan substitute)
- Salt and pepper to taste
- Olive oil for cooking

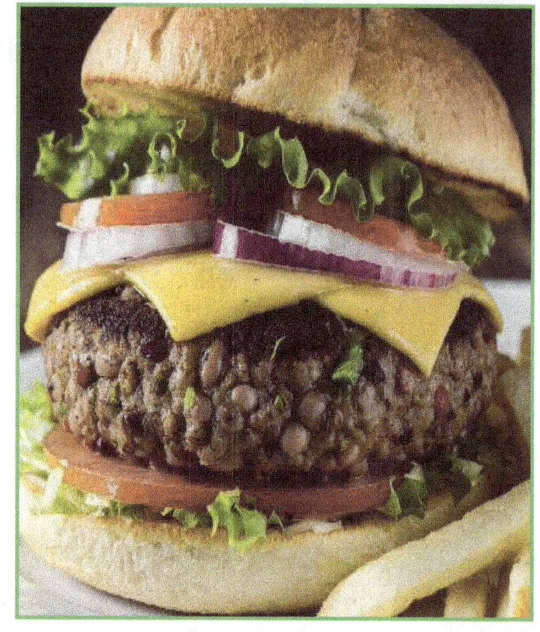

Directions:

1. In a big mixing container, pound the black beans using a fork or potato masher until almost smooth.
2. Add cooked quinoa, diced bell peppers, grated zucchini, diced red onion, minced garlic, ground cumin, smoked paprika, breadcrumbs, egg (or flaxseed meal), salt, and pepper to the mashed beans.
3. Mix everything until well combined and the mixture holds together.
4. Divide the mixture into equal portions and shape into burger patties.
5. Heat olive oil in a skillet over medium heat.
6. Cook the bean and vegetable burgers for about 4-5 minutes per side or until golden brown and cooked through.
7. Serve the homemade burgers on whole grain buns with your favorite toppings like lettuce, tomato slices, avocado, and mustard.

Nutritional information:

Calories: 250

Protein: 12g

Carbohydrates: 35g

Fiber: 10g

Fat: 8g

Ingredients:

- 1 medium head of cauliflower
- 1 tablespoon of olive oil
- 1 cup of sliced veggies mixture of (bell peppers, carrots, peas)
- 2 cloves of garlic, chopped
- 2 eggs, beaten
- 2 tablespoons soy sauce (or tamari for gluten-free)
- 1 teaspoon sesame oil
- Salt and pepper to taste
- Chopped green onions for garnish

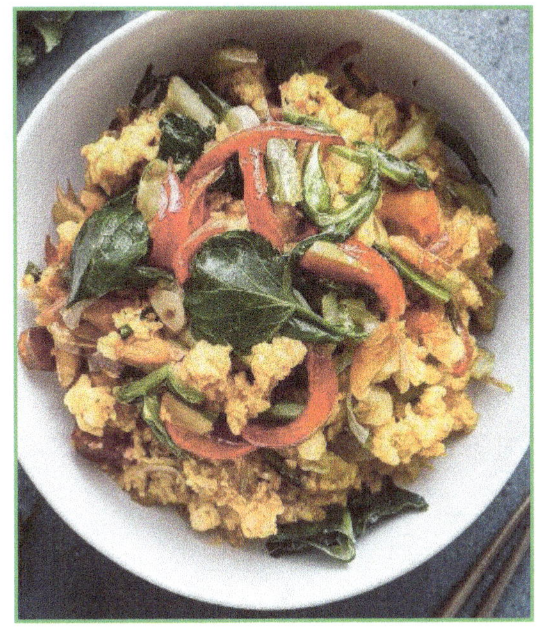

Directions:

1. Chop the cauliflower into pieces and pulse in a food processor until the texture resembles rice.
2. Heat olive oil in a big saucepan with medium heat.
3. Add minced garlic and diced mixed vegetables to the skillet. Stir-fry until vegetables are tender.
4. Push the vegetables to one side of the skillet and add beaten eggs to the other side. Scramble the eggs until cooked.
5. Mix all together in the saucepan.
6. Add cauliflower rice to the skillet, along with soy sauce, sesame oil, salt, and pepper.
7. Stir-fry for a few minutes until the cauliflower rice is heated through and well combined with the other ingredients.
8. Before serving, sprinkle with finely sliced green onion.

Nutritional information:

Calories: 180

Protein: 8g

Carbohydrates: 15g

Fiber: 6g

Fat: 10g

Ingredients:

- 2 acorn squashes, halved and seeds removed
- 1 cup of cooked quinoa
- 1 cup of cooked lentils
- 1 cup minced apples
- 1/4 cup chopped pecans
- 1/4 cup dried cranberries
- 2 tablespoons maple syrup
- 1 teaspoon ground cinnamon
- Salt and pepper to taste
- Olive oil for drizzling

Directions:

1. Preheat the oven to 375°F (190°C). Line the surface of a baking sheet with parchment paper.
2. Place acorn squash halves on the baking sheet, cut side up. Sprinkle with olive oil, then season with pepper and salt.
3. Roast squash in the preheated oven for about 30 minutes or until tender.
4. In a bowl, mix together cooked quinoa, cooked lentils, diced apples, chopped pecans, dried cranberries, maple syrup, ground cinnamon, salt, and pepper.
5. Stuff each roasted acorn squash half with the quinoa-lentil mixture.
6. Return stuffed squash to the oven and bake for an additional 10-15 minutes.
7. Serve the stuffed acorn squash hot as a nutritious meal.

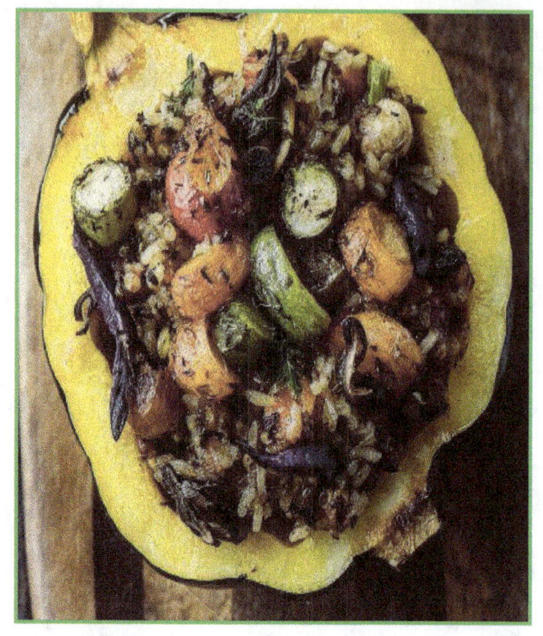

Nutritional information:

Calories: 320

Protein: 12g

Carbohydrates: 55g

Fiber: 12g

Fat: 8g

Ingredients:

- 1 medium spaghetti squash
- 1 pound of lean ground turkey
- 1/4 cup whole wheat breadcrumbs
- 1 egg
- 1/4 cup grated Parmesan cheese
- 2 cloves of garlic, minced it
- 1 teaspoon dried oregano
- 1 teaspoon dried basil
- Pepper and salt to enrich taste
- Marinara sauce (store-bought or homemade)
- Fresh basil leaves for garnish

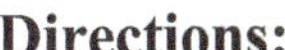

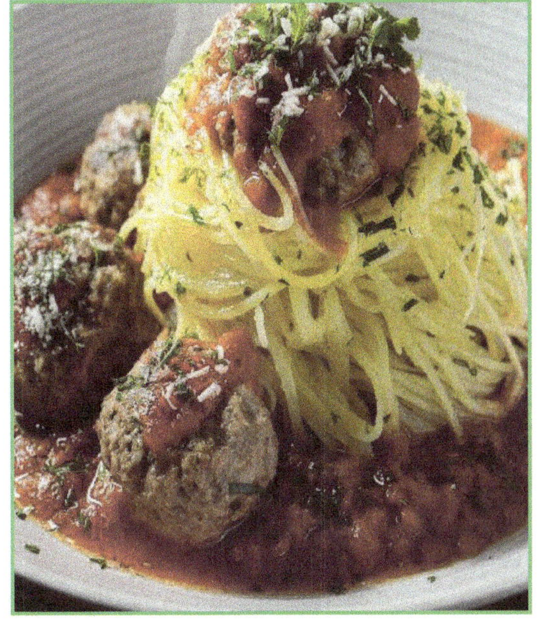

Directions:

1. Preheat the oven to 400°F (200°C) and line the baking surface with parchment paper.
2. Chop the spaghetti squash in half lengthwise and remove the seeds.
3. Place squash halves on the baking sheet, cut side down. Roast in a warm oven for 30-40 minutes, until tender.
4. While the squash is roasting, prepare the turkey meatballs. In a bowl, combine ground turkey, breadcrumbs, egg, grated Parmesan cheese, minced garlic, dried oregano, dried basil, salt, and pepper. Mix well and form into meatballs.
5. Heat a non-stick skillet over medium heat and cook the meatballs until browned and cooked through.
6. Heat marinara sauce in a separate pot.
7. Once the squash is cooked, use a fork to scrape the flesh into strands.
8. Serve the spaghetti squash topped with turkey meatballs and marinara sauce.
9. Sprinkle with freshly cut basil leaves prior to serving.

Nutritional information:

Calories: 350

Protein: 28g

Carbohydrates: 30g

Fiber: 6g

Fat: 12g

Ingredients:

- 1 cup of pearl barley, rinsed
- 6 cups vegetable broth
- 1 onion, chopped
- 2 carrots, diced
- 2 celery stalks, diced
- 1 cup of diced tomatoes
- 1 cup chopped spinach
- 1 teaspoon dried thyme
- 1 teaspoon dried rosemary
- Salt and pepper to taste
- Fresh parsley for garnish

Directions:

1. In a large pot, combine pearl barley and vegetable broth. Bring to a boil.

2. Reduce heat and simmer covered for about 30 minutes.

3. Add chopped onion, diced carrots, diced celery, diced tomatoes, dried thyme, dried rosemary, salt, and pepper to the pot.

4. Continue to simmer covered for another 20-25 minutes or until vegetables are tender and barley is cooked.

5. Stir in chopped spinach and cook for an additional 5 minutes.

6. Adjust seasoning if needed.

7. Serve the barley and vegetable soup hot, garnished with fresh parsley.

10.

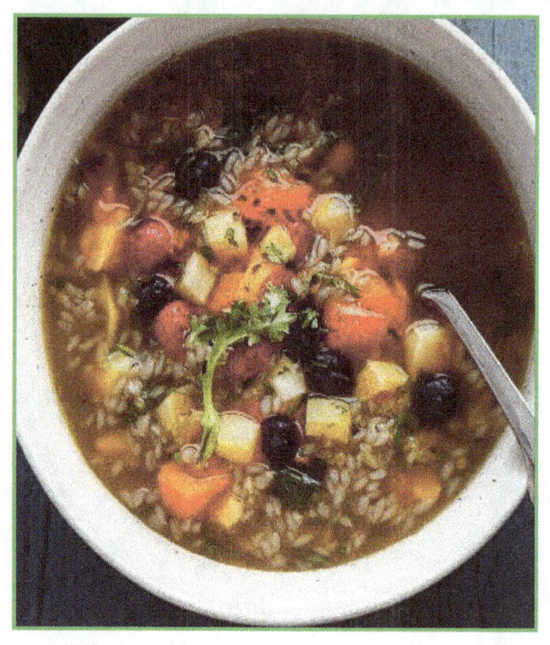

Nutritional information:

Calories: 280

Protein: 8g

Carbohydrates: 55g

Fiber: 12g

Fat: 2g

CHAPTER 7

SNACK IDEAS FOR DIVERTICULITIS DIET

GREEK YOGURT AND BERRY PARFAIT

Ingredients:

- 1 cup Greek yogurt (unsweetened)
- 1/2 cup of mixed berries (which include strawberries, blueberries, and raspberries)
- 2 tablespoons granola (choose a high-fiber variety)
- 1 tablespoon honey (optional)
- Salt and pepper to taste

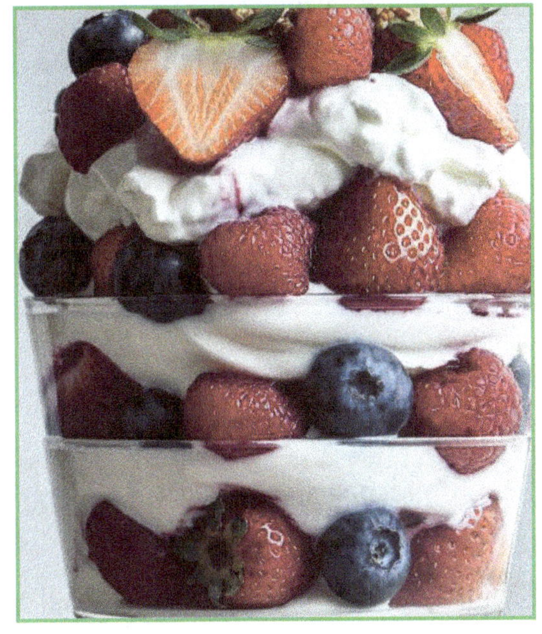

Directions:

1. In a glass or dish, combine the Greek yogurt, mixed berries, and granola together.
2. Drizzle honey or maple syrup on top if desired.
3. Repeat the layers if making multiple servings.
4. Serve chilled as a healthy and satisfying snack.

Nutritional information:

Calories: 200

Protein: 15g

Carbohydrates: 30g

Fiber: 5g

Fat: 5g

Ingredients:

- 1 cup of baby carrots
- 1 cup of slices cucumber
- 1 cup of bell pepper strips (any color)
- 1/2 cup cherry tomatoes
- 1/4 cup hummus (choose a low-fat variety)

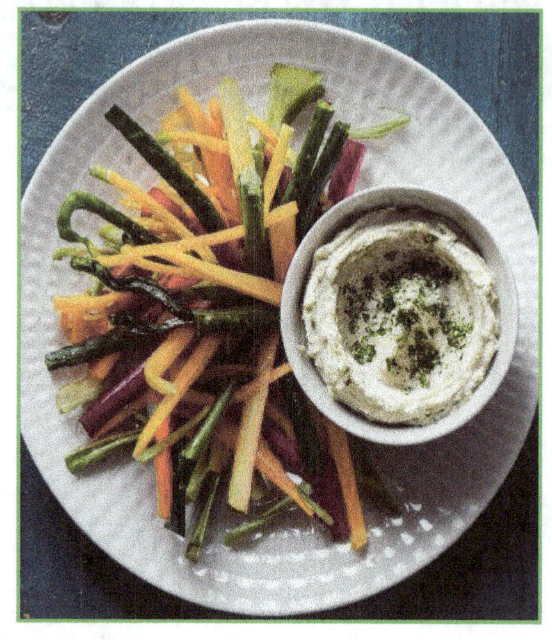

Directions:

1. Wash and prepare the vegetables by cutting them into sticks or slices.
2. Arrange the vegetable sticks and cherry tomatoes on a plate.
3. Serve with a side of hummus for dipping.
4. Enjoy this crunchy and nutritious snack.

Nutritional information:

Calories: 150

Protein: 5g

Carbohydrates: 20g

Fiber: 6g

Fat: 6g

Ingredients:

- 1 medium apple and slice it
- 2 tablespoons almond butter (unsweetened)

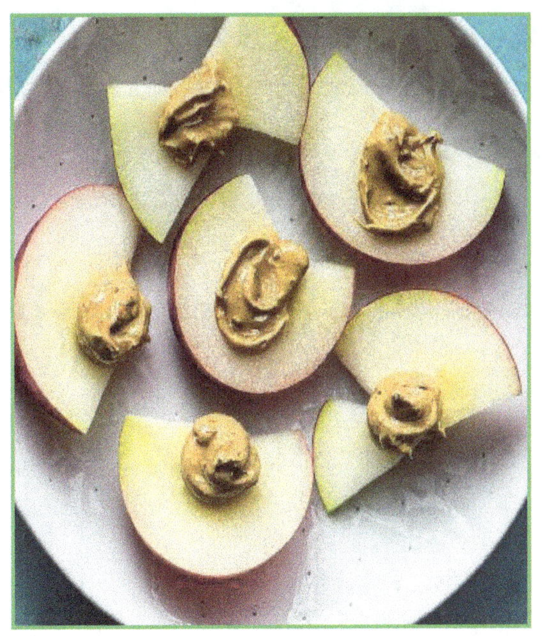

Directions:

1. Wash and core the apple, then slice it into wedges.
2. Spread the almond butter over each apple slice.
3. Arrange the apple slices on a plate.
4. This snack is rich in fiber and healthy fats.

Nutritional information:

Calories: 200

Protein: 4g

Carbohydrates: 25g

Fiber: 7g

Fat: 11g

Ingredients:

- 6 whole grain crackers (choose a high-fiber brand)
- 1/2 cup low-fat cottage cheese
- 1/2 avocado, sliced
- Sprinkle of black pepper and paprika (optional)

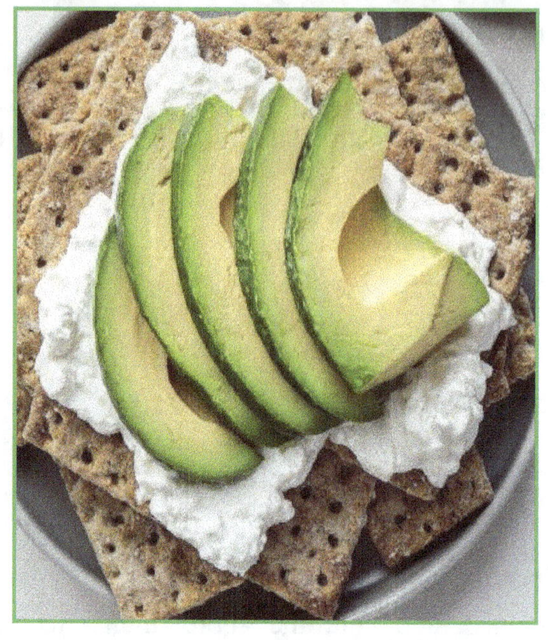

Directions:

1. Spread cottage cheese evenly on the whole grain crackers.
2. Top each cracker with a slice of avocado.
3. Sprinkle with black pepper and paprika if desired.
4. Serve this creamy and satisfying snack.

Nutritional information:

Calories: 220

Protein: 10g

Carbohydrates: 20g

Fiber: 5g

Fat: 10g

Ingredients:

- 1/4 cup almonds
- 1/4 cup walnuts
- 1/4 cup pumpkin seeds
- 1/4 cup dried cranberries (unsweetened)
- 1/4 cup dark chocolate chips (optional)

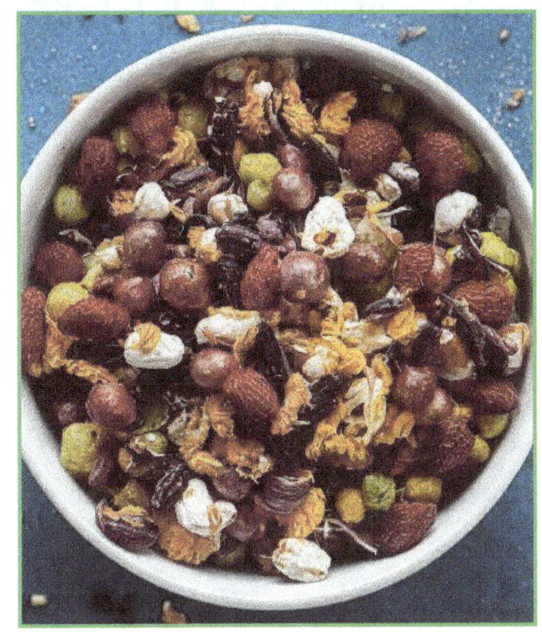

Directions:

1. In a bowl, combine almonds, walnuts, pumpkin seeds, dried cranberries, and dark chocolate chips.
2. Mix well to distribute the ingredients evenly.
3. Portion out the trail mix into snack-sized bags for convenient grab-and-go snacks.
4. Enjoy the mix of crunchy nuts and sweet dried fruits.

Nutritional information:

Calories: 250

Protein: 8g

Carbohydrates: 20g

Fiber: 5g

Fat: 18g

These snack choices contain a variety of vitamins, including fiber, protein, and healthy fats, which are essential to a diverticulitis diet.

Adjust component sizes to suit your dietary needs.

CHAPTER 8

TIPS FOR DINING OUT WITH DIVERTICULITIS

When choosing diverticulitis-friendly restaurants can significantly improve your eating experience when coping with this ailment. Here are some pointers to keep in mind when dining out:

1. Menu Variety: Look for restaurants that have a diverse selection of foods, including as fresh fruits and vegetables, lean proteins, and healthy grains. A broad menu ensures that you can find appropriate items that are compatible with your diverticulitis-friendly diet.

2. Ingredient Transparency: Select eateries that are open about their ingredients and processing procedures. This information allows you to make more informed decisions and avoid foods that may cause pain for your diverticulitis condition, such as processed meats, spicy dishes, or high-fat foods.

3. Customization Options: Choose restaurants that allow you to customize your own food. This allows you to request substitutions such as steamed vegetables instead of fried, whole grain alternatives instead of refined grains, or sauces and dressings on the side to have more control over your meal.

4. Fresh and Natural Foods: Choose eateries that use fresh, natural ingredients in their cuisine. Freshly made meals are frequently easier on the digestive system and contain less chemicals or preservatives, which can irritate diverticulitis.

5. Friendly and accommodating staff: Look for eateries that are willing to fulfill dietary restrictions. Informing the server of your illness and dietary preferences can assist them in recommending appropriate menu options or alterations.

6. Portion Sizes: Pay attention to the portion sizes provided by the restaurant. Choose smaller servings or split larger dishes to avoid overeating, which can strain the digestive tract and potentially cause diverticulitis symptoms.

7. Hydration Options: Choose a restaurant that serves hydrating beverages like water, herbal teas, or freshly squeezed juices. Maintaining proper hydration is critical for gut health and can improve overall wellbeing.

8. Comfortable Ambiance: Select restaurants that provide a comfortable and peaceful ambiance in which you may enjoy your lunch without worry or discomfort. A good dining atmosphere can help you digest better and enjoy your meal more.

By keeping these tips in mind and communicating your dietary needs with restaurant staff, it will make your dining out with diverticulitis a more enjoyable and manageable experience.

CONCLUSION

This book **"Diverticulitis Cookbook"**, is a whole guide on managing diverticulitis by paying concerted attention to what we eat and healthy lifestyle choices. Key points covered in this book include:

- Highlighting dietary aspects of high-fiber foods like fruits, vegetables, whole grains and legumes to aid digestion.

- Identifying trigger foods that cause symptoms and having skills on handling the same.

- Understanding when one should see a doctor for treatment recommendations.

- Utilizing tips on meal planning as well as cooking recipes tailored for people with diverticulitis.

Adopting a healthy way of living does not end at eating only; it involves exercising regularly, stress reduction techniques, proper hydration and enough sleep. This way, our lives become better off giving us an opportunity to improve our general body wellness too.

But also, for the digestive wellness journey you're on remember that small changes lead to enormous improvements over time. Thus heed your body's words do not take chances with its health.

Finally, this **"Diverticulitis Cookbook"** aims to provide you with useful resources, knowledge, and proposals to help you scape through the problems of diverticulitis while still enjoying a fulfilling and delectable culinary experience. Here is to your fitness and happiness on this nourishing journey ahead.

Here are some tips for prepping and storing your meals, especially if you are a busy person:

1. Plan Ahead: Take a while each week to plot your food. Create a menu for the approaching days, together with breakfast, lunch, dinner, and snacks. This plans will help you live prepared and make sure you have got diverticulitis-pleasant options effortlessly to be had.

2. Batch Cooking: Consider batch cooking larger portions of meals that can be portioned out and stored for later use. For example, put together a big pot of vegetable soup, a batch of whole grain pasta salad, or grilled hen breasts that can be integrated into numerous dishes for the duration of the week.

3. Use Storage Containers: Invest in appropriate high-quality, hermetic storage packing containers that are microwave-safe and freezer-friendly. Portion out your food into these containers, making it smooth to seize a pre-made meal while you're brief on time.

4. Label and Date: When storing food inside the fridge or freezer, make sure to label every container with the contents and date of training. This will help you maintain song of freshness and make sure you are ingesting meals before they spoil.

5. Freeze in Portions: If you are batch cooking, freeze food in character or own family-sized portions. This way, you can defrost and reheat simplest what you need, decreasing meals waste and making sure each meal is sparkling.

6. Pre-cut Ingredients: Save time all through meal prep by way of pre-cutting greens, culmination, and proteins. Store these prepped substances in separate bins within the refrigerator, so they're equipped for use while cooking.

7. Stock Healthy Staples: Keep your pantry and refrigerator stocked with wholesome staples like canned beans, entire grains, frozen greens, low-sodium broths, and lean proteins. These substances may be mixed quickly to create nutritious meals in a pinch.

8. Utilize Slow Cookers and Instant Pots: This kitchen home equipment are lifesavers for busy schedules. You can installation substances in the morning and come home to a delicious, ready-to-eat meal in the night without an awful lot effort.

9. Pre-component Snacks: Prepare grab-and-cross snacks like reduce-up end result, yogurt cups, combined nuts, or whole grain crackers with hummus. Having these healthy snacks easily available can prevent you from accomplishing for much less nutritious options whilst starvation moves.

10. Rotate and Refresh: Periodically rotate your meal alternatives and refresh your menu to keep away from monotony. Experiment with new recipes, flavors, and ingredients to hold your meals thrilling and fun.

By following these meal prep and storage tips, you can make healthy eating more convenient and sustainable, even with your busy schedule. These practices not only save time but also support your diverticulitis-friendly diet goals.

I will love your observation and honest review on this book for me to make other publications better.

If you have any further questions related to the book or relate to personal health, just know you have made a new friend to share your feelings with and I promise to be responsive and give you advice to the best of my knowledge, so you can contact me through this email: CarolynShart1@gmail.com

Could you please leave us a review? Your honest review is not only priceless but crucial in helping our future endeavors.

By leaving a review, you not only help us understand what resonates with you but also empower fellow readers to make informed decisions and help this book reach more potential readers. Your words have the power to inspire and guide others, creating a community of shared insights and connections. Together, let's celebrate the joy of meaningful communication and the beauty of heartfelt gestures.

Thank you for being a valuable reader and we look forward to hearing from you.

Kindly open your phone camera and place it on the barcode to scan. It will link you directly to the review page.

Very seamless.

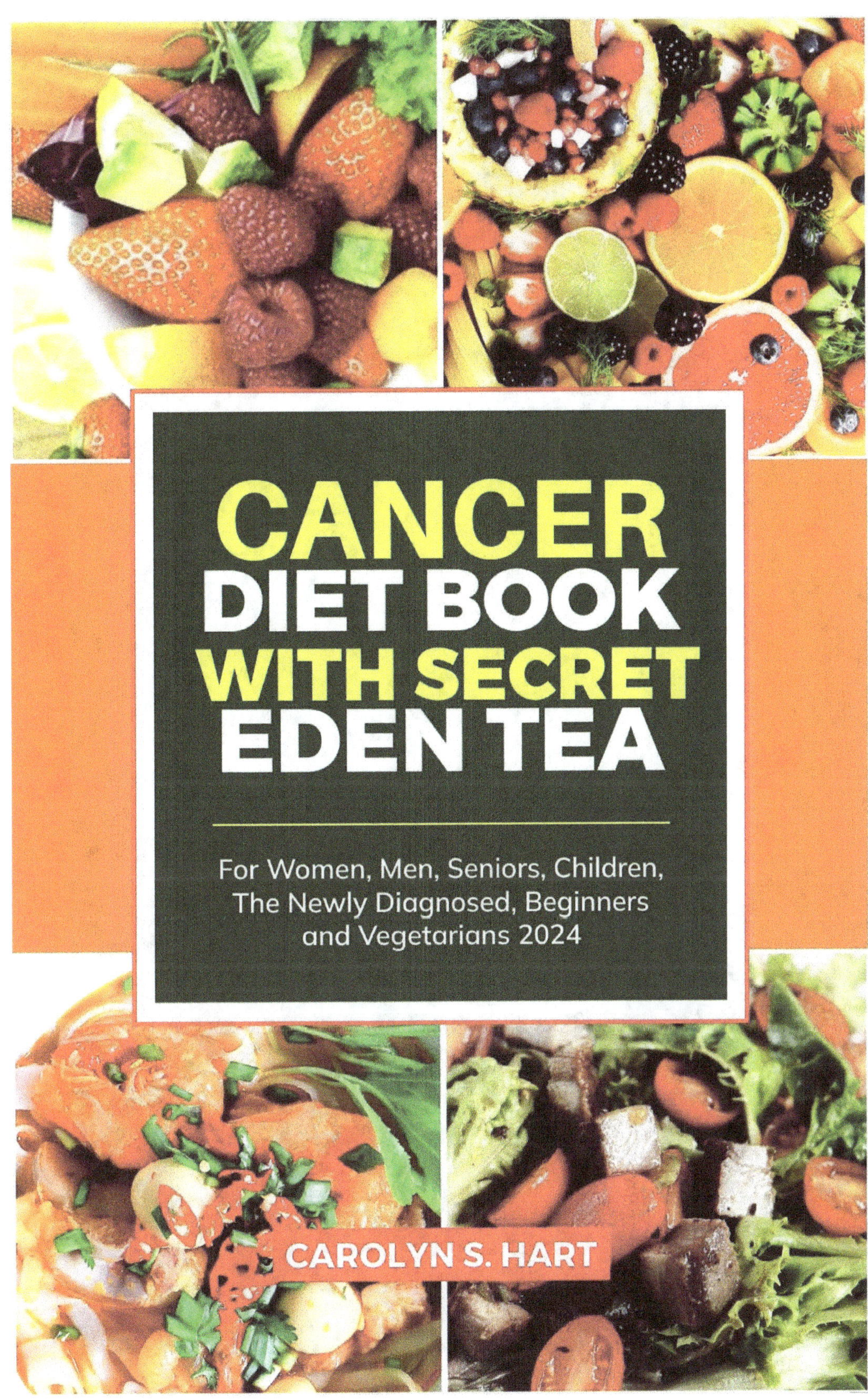

CANCER
DIET BOOK
WITH SECRET
EDEN TEA

For Women, Men, Seniors, Children,
The Newly Diagnosed, Beginners
and Vegetarians 2024

CAROLYN S. HART

LUNG CANCER

DIET COOKBOOK

OVER
1840
RECIPE

WITH NUTRITIONAL NEED WHOLE-FOOD RECIPES
TREATMENT TO OPTIMIZE LUNG CANCER TREATMENT
AND RECOVERY

CAROLYN S. HART